STD
CASE MANAGEMENT

INTERNATIONAL ENCYCLOPAEDIA OF AIDS-7

STD
CASE MANAGEMENT

Editor
Dr. Digumarti Bhaskara Rao
M.Sc., M.A., M.A., M.Ed., Ph.D.
R. V. R. College of Education
Guntur–522 006
Andhra Pradesh. (INDIA)

2000
DISCOVERY PUBLISHING HOUSE
NEW DELHI-110 002

First Published-2000

ISBN 81-7141-529-6

Published by:
DISCOVERY PUBLISHING HOUSE
4831/24, Ansari Road, Prahlad Street,
Darya Ganj, New Delhi-110 002 (*INDIA*)
Phone: 3279245
Fax: 91-11-3253475

Printed at:
Arora Offset Press
Laxmi Nagar, Delhi 110 092.

PREFACE

The HIV/AIDS is a new phenomenon in the human society. HIV destroys the immune system of human individuals, producing a defenselessness fatal state known as AIDS. The World Health Organisation has estimated that already one in every two hundred and fifty adults in the world is infected with Human Immunodeficiency Virus and according to WHO's projections a total of forty million men women and children worldwide will have been infected with HIV by the turn of this twentieth century. Visualising the devastating effects of the HIV/AIDS epidemic within our life times and beyond is difficult. Probably, no other disease in recent times has had the impact on human society generated by HIV/AIDS.

The HIV/AIDS epidemic has brought into focus many health related ethical, legal and human rights issues. This epidemic requires immediate and effective responses in new programming areas: attitudinal and behavioural changes, community-based care and support initiatives, and the maintenance of human development in the face of increasing rates of illness and deaths. At this point, education enters the scene as it can alter the HIV/AIDS situation since it brings change in the behaviour of the people.

This *International Encyclopaedia of AIDS* presents the worldwide information about HIV/AIDS, issues and challenges, reports and reviews, ethics laws and human rights, and educational activities and programmes to keep the policy makers, planners, professionals, activists, researchers, educationists, teachers and students well informed of the epidemic.

Dr. Digumarti Bhaskara Rao
26 January 1999
The Republic Day of India

ACKNOWLEDGEMENT

I am thankful to the World Health Organisation and its associated offices for using their material namely School Health Education to prevent AIDS and STD: A Resource Package for Curriculum Planners-Handbook for Curriculum Planners. Student's Activities, Teachers' Guide, Global Programme on AIDS-HIV Prevention and Care: Teaching Modules for Nurses and Midwives, Global Programme on AIDS. Community HIV Prevention Handbook; STD care Management-workbooks 1-7, Facing the Challenge of HIV/AIDS/STDs: A Gender-based Response; HIV/AIDS and STD surveillance Data Management and Use-Report, Bangkok, 1995; Carrying out HIV Sentinal Surveillance-A Guide for Programme Managers, AIDS Prevention and Care in the workplace: Enhancing the Role of Private Sector; HIV Testing Policies and Guidelines; Carrying out HIV Sentinel surveillance; AIDS Prevention; Understanding and Living with AIDS; AIDS: A Modern Epidemic; HIV/AIDS in South-East Asia: IXth meeting of the National Programme Managers, New Delhi, 1993; Information, Education and Communication: A Guide for AIDS Programme Managers, Handbook on AIDS Home Care; HIV/AIDS in South-East Asia: A Pictorial summary; etc.

I am thankful to the United Nations Development Programme, UNDP's HIV and Development Programme, and UNDP's Regional Projects on HIV and Development for using their material namely Economic Implications of AIDS in Asia; Socio Economic Implications of the Epidemic; NGOs Working with Sex workers; NGO Responses to HIV/AIDS in Asia-Case Studies; HIV in the Workplace: Dealing with the Issues-Role Plays, Development and the HIV Epidemic, Law Ethics and HIV; HIV Law and Law Reform; Issue Papers; Study Papers; Working Papers; etc.

I am thankful to the Health and Nutrition Centre, Republic of Philippines for using its material namely sourcebook on HIV/AIDS Prevention Education for Tertiary Educational Institutions.

I am thankful to the Curriculum Development Programme, Ministry of Education, Government of Thailand for using its material namely Institutional Modules for AIDS Education.

I am thankful to US Department of Health and Human Services: Whitman-Walker Clinic, Inc., USA; East-West Centre, USA; National AIDS Control Organisation, Government of India; Academy of Culture Communication Education Science and Service, Guntur, United Nations and its agencies for using their material.

I am grateful to Bhaskar Bhattacharji; V. Alexeev, Geeta Sethi, Elizabeth Reid, Mina Mauerstein-Bail, A. A. Trinidad, Palomi Cuchi, D. Pushpa Latha for their kind co-operation.

Dr. Digumarti Bhaskara Rao,
Secretary
ACCESS
D-43, S.V. N. Colony,
Guntur-522 006

CONTENTS

1

INTRODUCTION TO STD CASE MANAGEMENT

Welcome to this training programme. You have been chosen to participate in a fresh approach to the challenging task of managing cases of sexually transmitted diseases (STD).

This approach includes the syndromic management of STD, using flow-charts. It offers many benefits, as you will discover during your study. One of these benefits is that with syndromic management, all trained first-line service providers can diagnose and treat patients with an STD 'on the spot'.

STD are a very common and serious problem in the world. Although there are more than 20 kinds of organisms which can spread through sex, these different STD tend to cause similar symptoms and signs. For example, discharge from the penis (urethra) or vagina, and genital ulcer are common STD symptoms and signs. We call each set of symptoms/signs a syndrome. In the table below are some of the common syndromes and the STD which cause them:

Syndromes and the STD causing them

Syndrome	Cause of STD
Urethral discharge	Gonorrhoea Chlomydiol infection
Vaginal discharge	Trichomoniasis Bacterial vaginosis Candidiasis Gonorrhoea Chlamydiol infection

{Cont.}

Ulcer/s	Syphilis Chancroid Donovosis
Lower abdominal pain	Gonorrhoea Chlomydiol infection Anaerobic bacteria

As you can see, each syndrome has several causes. To tell which organism is causing a particular syndrome requires a laboratory to which most health workers and patients with STD don't have easy access. This is why WHO recommends syndromic case management of STD. This means that when a patient has a particular syndrome you should treat him/her for all the common STD causing this syndrome. It also means learning how to communicate with patients, providing them with the essential information they need, and managing their sexual partners.

It is not important to remember the names of all STD listed in the table - it is more important to learn how to diagnose and manage each syndrome. These workbooks teach you about syndromic case management, using flow-chorts. You will learn how to manage the syndromes listed above, as well as a few others.

Whatever your role is or will be in STD case management, this training progromme will equip you with the information and skills you need. It will help you to:

- appreciate the problem of STD throughout the world;
- identify the features of a syndromic approach to diagnosis and treatment of STD;
- develop your skills in interviewing, history-taking and diagnosis;
- use the seven syndromic flow-charts to help you disgnose and treat a patient with an STD;
- educate and motivate patients about the prevention and successful treatment of STD, including the importance of following treatment instructions and engaging in safe sex;
- treat the partners of patients who attend your health centre;
- consider the value of recording the number of STD cases you see in the course of your work, and how you and others might use such information.

This Programme Introduction will introduce you to the workbooks and help you to identify your learning needs, based upon the role you will play in STD case management. It will also advise you on how to plan your study, whether you are studying with a group of people or mainly on your own.

About the workbooks

The STD Case Management programme is comprised of seven workbooks. Below 15 a short description of each one.

1. The Transmission and Control of STD introduces you to the size and scope of the epidemic of sexually transmitted diseases. You will learn why STD place a major burden on individuals, families, health services and national economies.
2. Using Flow-chorts for Syndromic Management explains the problems of the classic approaches to STD case management, and introduces the syndromic approach as an altern ıtive. You will explore how syndromic case management can be effective in treating and preventing STD and learn how the flow-charts work.
3. History-taking and Examination takes you step-by-step through what to ask. how to ask it and how to examine patients.
4. Diagnoses and Treatment takes you step-by-step through each of the syndromic flow-charts. It includes the specific signs and symptoms to help make a diagnosis, as well as a list of drugs recommended by WHO for each condition identified.
5. Educating the Patient explores how to educate and motivate patients about STD prevention and treatment by using effective education and interviewing skills.
6. Partner Management is about managing and treating a patient's sexual partners. This workbook describes two approaches to partner management and why it is so important that partners are treated.
7. Recording explores the benefits of gathering information about STD, both nationally or regionally and at your health centre. More complete statistics are urgently needed that give a fuller picture of the epidemiology of STD all over the developing world. If your health centre is planning to record the number of cases you see, the workbook will also give you sample recording sheets to practice with.

How to use the workbooks

The workbooks are so-called because they are just that: books that ask you to think, make notes, answer questions and work on projects.

The purpose of the activities is to help you reflect on your learning and check your understanding of key points as you study. In other words, they are an aid to effective learning.

Throughout each workbook you will find question and activity symbols like these.

This means there is a question for you to answer, usually by making notes. If the question has a number, you will find our answer to it at the back of the workbook - but don't read it until you've tried to answer the question yourself.

Most activities will ask you to either:

- *discuss something with colleagues or fellow learners, or*
- relate ideas or examples to local conditions or your own experience.

At the back of each workbook you will find a Review and an Action Plan or Project. The Action Plan suggests a way for you to develop practical skills before working with real patients.

To become competent in the main skills in syndromic case management of STD, it is also essential that you practise certain skills with colleagues or fellow learners. Where this is the case, the Action Plan contains careful guidance on how to make your practice as effective as possible.

You will also find a Glossary at the back of each workbook, to help you check any words with which you are not familiar.

Identifying your learning needs

These are the five steps in STD case management:

1. History-taking and examination.
2. Syndromic diagnosis and treatment, using flow-charts.
3. Education on safe sex, including condom promotion and provision.
4. Partner management.
5. Data gathering (recordings).

Some health centres have staff with specialist roles, who work with patients on specific aspects of their health - such as patient educators for example. In others each service provider works through every step with each STD patient. So, if you are not already sure of your role in syndromic management, you need to find out what it will be.

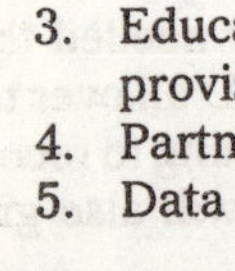

To clarify your role in syndromic case management, please consult your supervisor or trainer to find out which of the above steps will be your responsibility. Note them down below.:

Note down any skills or experience you have that may help you to carry out your responsibilities in syndromic case management of STD (history taking or conducting patient education sessions, for example).

If you feel that none of your current skills or experience are relevant to syndromic management, please don't worry - the workbooks will help you.

Please also remember that, even if you are very experienced - either in the usual approaches to STD case management or in a particular skill such as patient education - it is still essential to study the relevant workbooks carefully. You will need to know how to apply your skills or knowledge in the context of syndromic case management.

The matrix below shows how each workbook relates to the five steps in STD case management. Please tick the box beside each workbook you intend to study. (If possible, please study Workbooks 1 and 2 in any case. These will give you an overall understanding of how syndromic case management works, and how your role fits in to it.)

Tick	*Workbook Number*	*Steps in Case Management*
	1. The Transmission and Control of STD/HIV	None: an introduction to the burden of STD/HIV and the challenge of controlling them
	2. Using Flow-charts for Syndromic Management	None, but a useful introduction to syndromic case management
	3. History-Taking and Examination	Step 1: History-Taking and Examination
	4. Diagnosis and Treatment	Step 2: Use of syndromic flow charts to diagnose and treat for STD.
	5. Educating the Patient	Step 3: Education
	6. Partner Management	Step 4: Partner Management
	7. Recording	Step 5: Recording Data

Note: The next seven chapter in this part are the seven workbooks of this STD case Management Programme.

Planning how you will study

Ifs you are new to this sort of workbook, we hope you will find its approach to learning stimulating and helpful. Worldwide, learning like this is becoming accepted as at least as good as conventional training, and often better. Why? Because Iearners work at their own pace, they work at what they want to learn and also where and when they want to. We hope you too will en joy this form of study.

Studying with a group of people

If you are to study the workbooks as part of an organised course, with a tutor and a group of learners, then your tutor will guide you through the Action Plans and development activities. He or she will also lead discussions on many of the activities and questions.

You may be asked to read a whole or part of a workbook on your own, before coming together with your group or tutor to discuss issues or practice key skills. The workbook is a very flexible tool for this purpose, because you can make notes in it as you wish. If you are a fast reader, you can spend more time on the activities; if you read more slowly, nothing is lost because you can take what remains of the 'lesson' away to finish at your leisure!

Studying on your own

If you need to study one or more of the workbooks in your own time, it is very important that you answer each question and activity carefully, and that you check your answers to questions with the comments at the back of the workbook.

However, to learn effectively, discussion with others is also useful. You can work with other people from time to time: a trainer or supervisor and a small group of colleagues - preferably who are also studying this programme.

It is essential that you practise certain skills with one or two other people who are either learning or have experience in the appropriate step in syndromic case management of STD. The Action Plans for Workbooks 3, 5 and 6 suggest that you practice the appropriate skills in this way; they offer careful guidance on how to orgonise the practice in order to get as much as you can out of it.

Its is also useful to have someone to discuss your progress with someone you can turn to for support if you are studying on your own. Please ask your supervisor or a colleague experienced in syndromic management if they would be willing to support you in your learning.

ACTIVITY

Who might support you as you study?

With whom might you practice key skills and debate questions?

Extra study tips

- Find out when you will meet your tutor or ahead any training sessions. Ask which work books ,if any, you need to study before the meeting.
- If possible, make sure that you have a good place to study: preferably somewhere quiet where you will not be interrupted. If this is difficult to arrange, perhaps your tutor or supervisor can help you.
- It is also a good idea to make a study timetable: plan short study sessions that fit in with your working day. Try to study when you feel fresh and alert you won't learn so well when you are tired. For the same reason, three of four short sessions spread over a week are better than one whole day.
- Keep a note of any questions or problems as you study, and try to get answers or sort them out as soon as possible.

Remember: Use your tutor and colleagues: they are there to help you!

Best wishes with your learning!

2

THE TRANSMISSION AND CONTROL OF STD/HIV

A. INTRODUCTION

Sexually transmitted diseases (STD) are very common. The most widely known are gonorrhoea, syphilis and AIDS but there are more than 20 others. WHO, in 1995, estimates that every year there are more than 330 million new cases of curable STD. About 1 million infections are occurring every day.

This first workbook will help you to appreciate the extent of the problem that STD pose: a problem so severe that it ranks as a major epidemic.

The workbook will give you much of the information you need to appreciate the severity and impact of the epidemic. You will learn how STD are transmitted, what biological and social factors influence their transmission, their epidemiology and social and behovioural impact, and how STD facilitate the transmission of HIV-infection. Finally, you will learn why STD control is so difficult, and ways to improve it.

At the end of the workbook there is a project to help you learn about STD locally.

Your learning objectives

This workbook wills enable you to:

- identify how STD are transmitted and the factors that influence transmission;
- appreciate the serious complications that can arise from untreated STD;
- explore the extent of STD, including issues that may mask the true burden;
- understand how STD are linked with the spread of HIV;
- explain why the control of STD is so difficult, and what must be done to achieve control.

B. STD–TRANSMISSION

In many developing countries throughout the world, sexually transmitted diseases (STD) rank among the top five conditions for which adults seek health care. These diseases are important for two reasons: because of their magnitude, and because of their potential for causing serious complications.

The advent of the human immunodeficiency virus (HIV), another sexually transmissible infection, has drawn attention to the urgent need for prevention and control of STD.

This first section will help you to answer three questions:

- how are STD transmitted?
- what types of behaviour increase the risk of transmission?
- what biological and social factors influence transmission?

How are STD transmitted?

As their name implies, the main mode of transmission of STD is through unprotected penetrative sexual intercourse (vaginal or anal). Other modes of transmission include:

- mother-to-child: during pregnancy (HIV and syphilis), at delivery (gonorrhoea and chlamydia) or after birth (HIV);
- transfusions or other contact with blood or blood-products (syphilis, HIV).

What behaviours influence transmission?

If the main mode of transmission of STD is through sex then the following factors increase risk of infection:

- a recent change of partner;
- having more than one sexual partners;
- having a partner who has other partners;
- having sex with 'casual' partners, commercial sex-workers or their clients (partners whose other contacts are not known and whose status in terms of STD is not known);
- continuing to have sex with symptoms of an STD;
- if you have an STD, not informing sexual partners that they need treatment.

Not using a condom in any of these situations exposes both partners to a seriously high risk of infection.

There are many reasons why people behave in ways which increase the transmission of STD. These are often referred to as social factors. Read through the list below, consider which ones might apply to patients in your region, and which ones have not been mentioned.

Social factors that influence transmission

- **Failure to follow 'safe sex' measures, such as using condoms**

There are many reasons why people fail to follow safe sex practices. Perhaps the most important ones include:

— lack of knowledge of safe sex;
— lack of access to affordable condoms;
— dislike of condoms;
— cultural and religious reasons;
— the fact that sexual practices are deeply rooted in the everyday life of people and their communities.

- **Delay in getting STD treatment**

To name just a few reasons why people may fail to get early treatment:

— women with STD often have no symptoms;
— appropriate health facilities may not be available or affordable,
— health facilities do not have the necessary drugs;
— people may prefer to try alternative health sources such as traditional healers first;
— the stigma so often attached to STD may lead people to hide what they feel is shameful, and so avoid seeking treatment unless the levels of pain overrides their resistance.

- **Not taking the full, prescribed course of treatment for STD**

Effective treatment is only possible if patients take the full prescribed course of treatment. Patients may fail to do this for a variety of reasons, including the cost of treatment, lack of health education, conviction that the treatment taken so far will work, or low opinion of the health clinic's service.

- **Failure to bring in sexual partners for treatment**

Stigma may also affect a patient's readiness to inform his or her partner and the partner's readiness to accept treatment.

Biological factors that influence transmission

Apart from behavioural and social factors, certain biological factors also increase transmission of STD.

- **Age**

The nature of the vaginal mucosa and cervical tissue in young women makes them very susceptible to infection. Young women are specially at risk in cultures where they marry or become sexually active during their early teenage years.

- **Gender**

STD are primarily transmitted to women through vaginal intercourse. It easier for a woman to be infected by a man than for a man to be infected by a women in this way. This is because women have a larger surface exposed (i.e. the vagina) during penetrative sex.

- **Circumcision**

Circumcised men are less likely to get an STD than uncircumcised men.

ACTIVITY

Please note down:

(a) Anything that surprised you as a factor that influence transmission:

(b) Any of these factors that could apply to patients in your region:

(c) Any other factors in your region that we have not included in our list:

C. STD–THE PROBLEM

Why is it so important to control STD?

In answering this question, we need to explore three issues: the complications caused by STD when patients are not treated effectively, the extent of STD in the population, and the links between STD and transmission of HIV.

By the end of the section you will be better able to:

- discuss the frequency and distribution of STD; identify the
- range of serious complications which some STD can cause;
- explain the links between STD and HIV.

You may already be familiar with the main consequences and

complications caused by different STD. If so, please regard the next two pages as a review of your knowledge.

The frequency and distribution of STD

First of all, we need to consider the epidemiology (the frequency and distribution of a disease in the population). In this part of the section, we will explore questions such as these:

- what is the extent of the STD problem in different parts of the world?
- what is the distribution of STD by age, sex and occupation?
- do the existing statistics provide an accurate picture of the extent of STD? Why or why not?
- what is the effect of STD on a society?

STD, including HIV, are caused by the same high-risk sexual behaviour. Having multiple partners and changing partners often are risky and expose people to STD.

What is the extent of STD?

Worldwide in 1995, the World Health Organization estimates that there are over 330 million new cases of curable STD*

Please read the report below, which is based on a number of studies from many countries. It suggests that prevalence rates of STD seem to be far higher in developing countries than in developed countries. Why does the author think this is true?

Sexually transmitted diseases are a major public health problem in both developed and developing countries, but prevalence rates apparently are far higher in developing countries, where STD treatment is less accessible. Among women, syphilis prevalence rates may be 10 to 100 times higher in developing countries; gonorrhea rates may be 10 to 15 times higher; and chlamydia rates may be 2 to 3 times higher. For example, the annual rate of new gonorrhea infections in large African cities is 3 000 to 10 000 per 100 000 population, or as many as one in every 10 people. By comparison, in the US the annual incidence of gonorrhea was 233 per 100 000 population in 1991, and in Sweden, about 30 per 100,000 in 1987.

Among developing regions STDs appear to be more common in Africa than in Asia or Latin America. In a {recent/review ... a median of 20% of women attending family planning, antenatal, or other clinics in Africa had trichomoniasis, for example, while the median prevalence in Asian studies was 11%, and in Latin American studies, 12%.

Controlling Sexually Transmitted Diseases
Population Reports, June 1993, Page 3.

---

* gonorrhoea, chlamydial infection, syphilis and trichomoniasis.

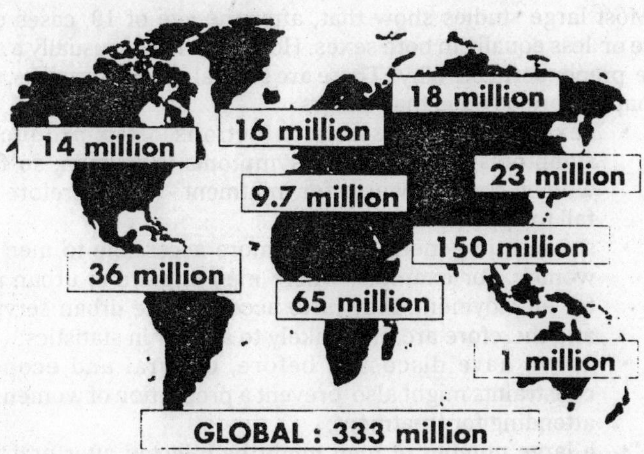

*Figure 1. Estimated new cases of curable STD * among adults, 1995.*

Throughout the article on the last page, you will find expressions such as 'apparently', 'may be' and 'appear to be'. These suggest that we need to be cautious about the evidence the figures suggest.

Who is affected?

STD, including HIV-infection, are widespread throughout the world. They affect sexually-active people of both sexes, so STD occur in both males and females. However, statistics rarely show an equal distribution between men and women nor do they show an equal distribution between different age groups.

Distribution of STD by age and sex

Most children below 14 years of age are free from infection. Other than for congenital syphilis, ophthalmia neonatorum and HIV-infection, most children under 14 years old are not affected by STD.

Between the ages of 14 and 19 years, cases occur more commonly among females. This is due to several factors:

- the start of sexual activity is usually earlier for girls than for boys;
- girls have sex with older partners, who are more experienced and also more likely to carry infections;
- biological vulnerability of young girls - due to characteristics of the genital tract of young girls, they are especially vulnerable to infection with STD.

For both males and females, rates of STD tend to be highest in the 15-30 age group, decreasing in later ages.

Most large studies show that, after the age of 19, cases occur more or less equally in both sexes. However, there is usually a slight male preponderance. Why? There are several possible reasons, some perhaps more obvious than others:

- sexually transmissible infections often produce no symptoms or only mild symptoms in women, so fewer women come forwards for treatment - and 'therefore' they fail to appear in statistics;
- services in general may be more accessible to men than women. For example, where men migrate to urban areas for employment, they have access to the urban services - and therefore are more likely to appear in statistics;
- as we have discussed before, cultural and economic constraints might also prevent a proportion of women from attending for treatment;
- a large number of men might be infected after practicing unsafe sex with small number of sex workers;
- older men may be more sexually active than women of the same age,
- men are more likely to change partners than women.

In many developing countries, the best available indicators of STD levels in women are surveys taken by antenatal, family planning, or gynaecological clinics. They show a high prevalence of STD among the women attending.

Vulnerable groups

In most communities there are certain people who may be particularly vulnerable to STD. These people vary from community to community but may include:

- teenage girls who are sexually active;
- women women who have several partners 'in order to make ends meet';
- commercial sex workers and their clients;
- men and women whose jobs force them to be away from their families or regular sexual partners for long periods of time.

For various reasons these people may seldom come to health facilities for treatment when they have an STD, and special efforts often need to be made to reach them.

How accurate can any figure be?

Most often, figures on STD are taken from the numbers attending health facilities for treatment. This tends to underestimate the true extent of STD in the general population for several reasons, some of which we have already covered:

- both men and women with STD may be symptom-free, but women more so than men. For example:
  - — 70% of women and 30% of men infected with chlamydia may not have symptoms;
  - — up to 80% of women and 10% of men infected with gonorrhoea may also not have symptoms;
- clinics offering treatment for STD may not be accessible to many of the population;
- many people with STD do not seek treatment, and in developing countries people are not routinely screened for STD when they seek other health care.
- because of the stigma attached to STD, many people seek treatment from alternative providers who do not report cases (such as traditional healers and pharmacists);
- some governments are reluctant to admit to a high prevalence of STD, although the AIDS epidemic is beginning to change this attitude.

The effect on society

The social and economic burden of STD is enormous. They place a heavy financial burden on families, communities and health services, which must devote much of their time to STD. In one African country more than 70% of the budget for antibiotic drugs was used for STD treatment. STD also reduce the productivity of men and women in what should be the prime of their lives. If the epidemic is not controlled, the loss to national incomes will be significant.

The complications of STD

You may already be familiar with the main consequences and complications of different STD. If so, please treat the next two pages as a review.

Recent evidence reveals that common STD contribute to the spread of AIDS. Persons with the STD listed below are more likely to become infected when exposed to HIV and are more likely to transmit HIV if they are infected with:

- gonorrhoea,
- chlamydia;
- syphilis;
- chancroid;
- trichomoniasis

STD can be devastating; in women they can be fatal. Complications include:

- chronic abdominal pain or infertility in women;
- potentially blinding eye infections or pneumonia in infants;
- death due to sepsis, ectopic pregnancy and cervical cancer;
- spontaneous abortion;
- Urethral stricture in men;
- infertility in men;
- there may be social consequences as well. For example, when a husband learns that his wife has an STD, the result can sometimes include beating or divorce. Husbands may abandon infertile wives.

Let's look at the consequences of the main STD in more detail.

Gonorrhoea and chlomydia are the main causes of pelvic inflammatory disease in women (PID is inflammation of the uterus, fallopian tubes, ovaries and sometimes the lower abdominal cavity). In fact, the pain of PID is often the first symptom that women with chlamydial infection notice, and at that point any damage to the fallopian tubes is irreversible. Chlamydia was relatively unknown 10 years ago. Even now, because laboratory confirmation is difficult, It is rarely diagnosed .

An article in Population Reports of 1993 stresses the link between PID and infertility in women:

PID and Infertility
Without treatment 55% to 85% of women with PID may become infertile
In a study in Zimbabwe 84% of 135 infertile women with abnormal fallopian tubes had a history of pelvic inflammatory disease....
Many women may lose their fertility without ever realizing that they had pelvic inflammatory disease. For example, in 14 studies of women with blocked fallopian tubes, 40% to 80% did not report that they had had pelvic inflammatory disease.

Controlling Sexually Transmitted Diseases
Population Reports, June 1993, Page 5.

Because PID permanently scars and narrows the fallopian tubes, it increases the, of risk of ectopic pregnancy - a condition that can be fatal to women. If the out-of place pregnancy causes the fallopian tube to rupture, there can be extensive haemorrhaging. Population Reports states that, in the developing world, ectop, pregnancy 'caused 1% to 5% of all maternal deaths'.

They add that:

Chlamydia and ectopic pregnancy
Pelvic inflammatory disease increases the risk that a pregnancy

will be ectopic by 7 to 10 - fold. A US study found that genital chlamydial infection more than doubled a woman's risk of having an ectopic pregnancy.

Controlling Sexually Transmitted Diseases
Population Reports, June 1993, Page 5.

In men, gonorrhoea and chlamydia can also lead to serious complications. An Infection can spread from the urethra (where it is known as urethritis) to the epididymis (where it is known as epididymitis). These complications can cause urethral stricture and infertility but they are rare nowadays.

Gonorrhoea and chlamydia in men
In men under age 35 the most common cause of epididymitis is gonorrheal or chlamydial infection. Before antibiotics became available. 10% to 30% of men had gonorrhea developed epididymitis, and 20% to 40% of men with epididymitis became infertile.

Controlling Sexually Transmitted Diseases,
Population Reports, June 1993, Page 5.

Gonorrhoea and chlamydia can also cause eye infections and pneumonia in babies.

Gonorrhoea and chlamydia in babies
In a number of developing countries ophthalmia neonatorum afflicts 5% of newborns. Without treatment ophthalmia neonatorum permanently damages the vision of 1% to 6% of affected infants. Chlamydia also may spread to the lungs of newborns and lead to chlamydial pneumonia.

Controlling Sexually Transmitted Diseases
Population Reports, June 1993, Page 5

Syphilis, in pregnancy can spread to the amniotic sac and infect the foetus. 40% of syphilitic pregnancies end in spontaneous abortion, stillbirth, or perinatal death.

Summary

Perhaps you find the extent of the complications quite shocking, even if you are an experienced service provider. It seems more shocking upon realizing that all these complications can be avoided if the correct treatment is provided sufficiently early. When we add HIV-infection, for which there is as yet no cure, and the knowledge that so many STD facilitate its transmission, we have a full picture of the outcomes of the STD epidemic.

So far, we have focused our discussion on all STD except for HIV, the human immunodeficiency virus and AIDS. That is the subject of the final part of this section.

The AIDS epidemic

HIV-infection, which causes AIDS, is spread by the same behaviour as other There is as yet no cure for AIDS, and it is fatal. We need to ask two quest about AIDS: first, what is the extent of this epidemic and, secondly, what links between the transmission of STD and HIV?

Table 1 shows the estimated, projected annual figures for HIV-infection by sex up to the year 2000, while Figure 2 shows the estimated distribution of total adult HIV-infections between the late 1970s/early 1980s and mid-1 995, continent by continent.

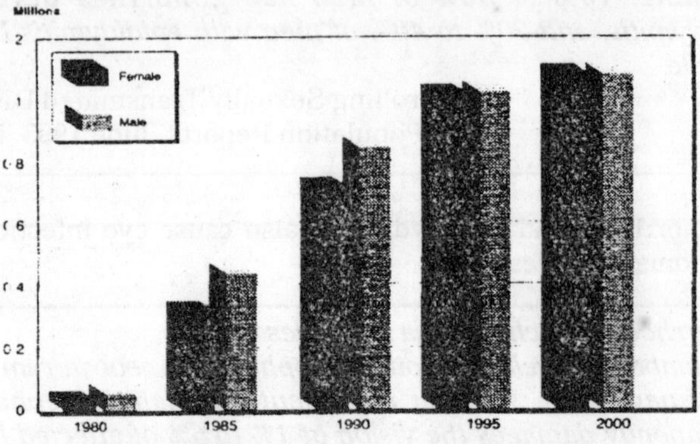

Table 1. Estimated /projected annual HIV-infections, by sex.

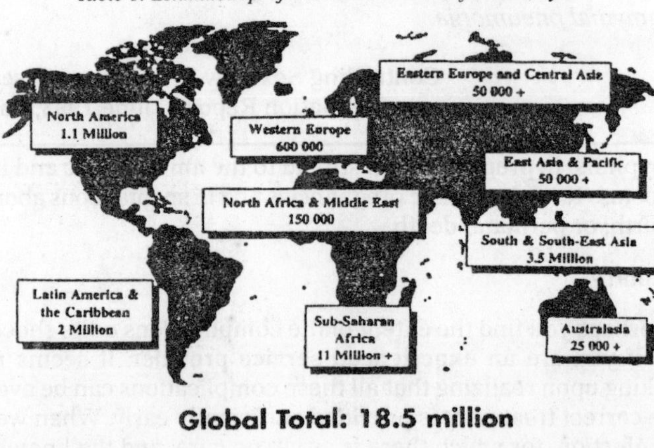

Figure 2. Estimated distribution of total adult HIV-infections from late 1970s/early 1980s until mid-1995.

By 1995, a total of 18.5 million adults and about 1.5 million children had been infected with HIV, according to World Health Organization estimates. In the year 2000 the projected annual figure for new cases of HIV-infection will be over 2 million, as Table 1 shows. By the same year, a total of 30 to 40 million) people will be infected. 10 million will have developed AIDS; 90% of the cases will be in developing countries.

These are conservative estimates but they confirm that AIDS is particularly serious in sub-Saharan Africa and South and South-East Asia, and a major epidemic throughout the world.

The link between STD and AIDS

As we have mentioned before, other sexually transmitted diseases make it easier for HIV to pass from one person to another. Chancroid, chlomydia, gonorrhoea, syphilis, and trichomoniasis may increase the risk of HIV transmission two to nine times. The link between HIV-infection and other STD may partly explain why HIV has spread so rapidly in Africa compared to Europe and the US, where STD are more often treated and cured.

The link is clearest between HIV-infection and STD that cause genital ulcers although not all studies have found an association:

Six of 10 studies in Kenya and Zaire, for example, found that people with genital ulcers, caused mainly by chancroid, were more likely to be infected with HIV than people without ulcers. Their risk was two to five times greater. Nine of 11 studies of syphilis and HIV-infection found an association. Syphilis increased the risk of HIV-infection threefold to ninefold for heterosexual men. Three of six studies of genital herpes and HIV-infection found an association. Herpes doubled the risk of HIV-infection for women and heterosexual men.

Controlling Sexually Transmitted Diseases
Population Reports, June 1993, Page 6

Do STD that don't cause ulcers increase the risk of HIV transmission?

Six studies found that chlamydia, gonorrhea, and trichomonissis, which do not cause ulcers, increase the risk of HIV transmission to women by three to five times. Several studies, however, have found no link between these STDs and HIV-infection, but methodological problems may have obscured the connection.

Controlling Sexually Transmitted Diseases,
Population Reports, June 1993, Page 6.

If the six studies referred to in the article are correct, then why do non ulcer-causing STD increase the risk of transmission of HIV?

These STDs may enhance HIV transmission because they increase the number of white blood cells - which are both targets and sources of HIV- the genital tract and because genital inflammation may cause microscopic cuts that can allow HIV to enter the body. Diseases causing vaginal and urethral inflammation are far more common than genital/ ulcer diseases and so may be responsible for a larger share of HIV transmission.

Controlling Sexually Transmitted Diseases
Population Reports, June 1993, Paged 6

To summarise the links between STD and HIV, we can say that STD increase the risk of HIV transmission. We could describe the risk in this way:

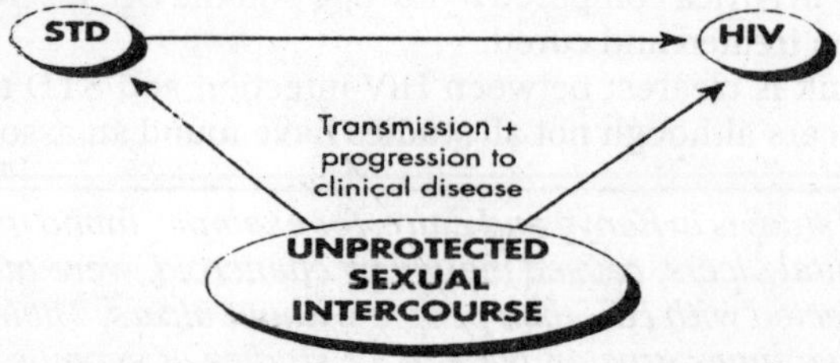

However it is also true that infection with HIV affects the other STD. How?

In people with HIV-infection other STDs may be more resistant to treatment. For example, several studies have reported that one-dose treatment for chancroid failed at least six times more often in HIV-infected patients than in patients without HIV-infection. Also, syphilis lesions may last longer in people infected with HIV, and these people may get gonorrhea more often. Thus HIV enhances its own transmission.

Controlling Sexually Transmitted Diseases,
Population Reports, June 1993, Page 6.

The article concludes with this point:

With longer-lasting STD symptoms, people with HIV-infection are more likely to transmit HIV and increase the pace of the AIDS epidemic.

Controlling Sexually Transmitted Diseases
Population Reports, June 1993, Page 6

So, we can develop the diagram above to show this two-way link between HIV and STD:

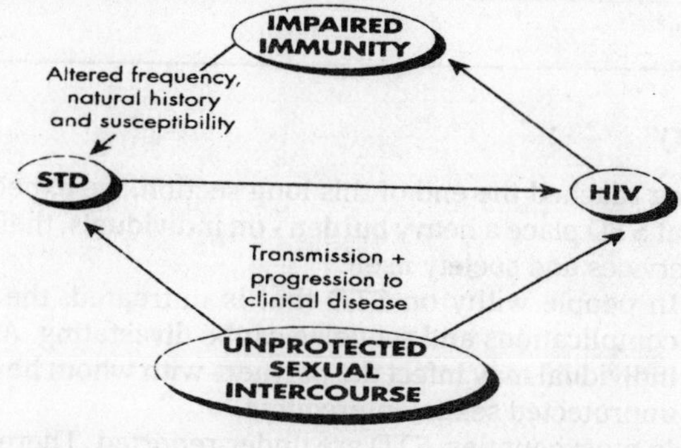

Figure 3. The interrelationship of STD and HIV-infection.

The exact link between STD and AIDS has not yet been fully worked out. However, treating people with STD provides a valuable opportunity for service providers to reach those at particularly high risk of acquiring AIDS.

QUESTION

If the link between HIV and other STD is new to you, try these questions in order to check your understanding.

1. *The extracts from the article on HIV and AIDS suggest that other STD increase the risk transmission of HIV. By how much? (Does it vary between STD?)*

2. *The article suggests that genital ulcers are a key cause of transmissibility, but that even those STD which do not cause ulcers may enhance transmission. HOW?*

____

____

____

3. How does HIV-infection affect transmission of other STD?

____

____

Summary

Having reached the end of this long section, we expect you will agree that STD place a heavy burden - on individuals, their families, health services and society itself.

- In people withy on STD that is untreated, the symptom complications and sequelae canbe divastating. An infected individual may infect the partners with whom he or she has unprotected sexual intercourse.
- In most counties, STD are under-reported. There are many more cases than are recorded.
- STD can cause serious compilations and death, having a serious impact on society. They affect productivity and incur considerable costs for individuals and health services.
- Among people who have unprotected sexual intercourse with many partners, STD spread quickly. In counties where seling sex is one of the few economic activities open to poor women, more women are put at risk.
- STD affect the outcomes of pregnancy and child birth. HIV and syphilis infects the baby before it is born, gonorrhoeo may infects the baby as its passes through the birth canal, chlamydia and gonorrhoea can make women infertile and result in ectopic pregnancy and chlamydia can cause infections in the new born.
- STD are linked the spread of AIDS. There is a strong link between having STD (especially genital ulcer and becoming HIV-positive. HIV-infection may make people more susceptible to other STD - and may make other STD more resistant to treatment.

ACTIVITY

At the back of this workbook, is an information gathering project. Meanwhile, you might like to consider the questions below. Please note down your thoughts and then discuss the questions with colleagues.

To your knowledge, what are the effects of STD on individuals and families in your region?

What are the health worker and community attitudes to people known to have an STD?

What health services, such as modern or traditional ones, might people with STD seek in your region? Why?

What happens to women who become infertile because of STD infection?

How aware are people in your community of safe-sex messages and the causes of STD including HIV?

D. THE CHALLENGE OF CONTROLLING STD

The goal of STD control is to reduce the spread of STD infection and to prevent more csses of STD. But control is difficult for a number of reasons.

QUESTION

What makes the control of STD so difficult? Consider what you have read so far and list as many factors as you can.

Compare your notes with what we have written on the next page.

In fact, many factors make the control of STD difficult. We have discussed some already, when listing the social and biological factors that influence transmission and the difficulty of obtaining accurate statistics. You would be quite right to have listed any of those factors. However, there are four additional factors that we would like to emphasise at this point.

It is difficult to change sexual behaviour

Any behavioural change is difficult. Knowledge does not always lead to a change in behaviour. The difficulty in controlling STD lies in the fact that sexual practices are deeply rooted in the everyday life and culture of people. Sexual behaviour is vital to who we are and how we feel about ourselves. It is shaped by culture and influenced by religion. Sexual behaviour, because it is very personal and deeply rooted, is thus very difficult to change.

The use of drugs, including alcohol, impairs people's ability to make good decisions, including taking protective measures against STD/HIV-infection.

Sex is embarrassing to discuss

Because sex is embarrassing to discuss, people may be too shy to ask for the information they need, slow to come for treatment and reluctant to tell their partners. Talking about sex can make us uncomfortable and may be taboo. As you know, this is a major reason why STD are often under-reported - and why it 15 often not recognized as a major primary health care problem. People often fee shame if they have, or suspect they have, an STD.

Many STD carriers have no symptoms

People with STD who are symptom-free can spread the disease without even knowing that they have it. This complicates treatment programmes because reaching these people requires complex interventions.

Treatment is not always simph - or effective

Finally, we need to mention the resistance of some bacteria, such as those causing gonorrhoea and chancroid, to antibiotics. Resistance to drugs requires changes in the drug of choice and use of increasingly expensive drugs to achieve control. For example, there used to be a simple, effective treatment for gonorrhoea; this is increasingly a problem because of the organism's resistance to penicillin. For viral STD such as HIV and herpes there is no effective treatment. The possibility of a vaccine for STD such as HIV does not seem very likely at this time as the virus is continually evolving.

So what can be done to control STD?

Please try answering the question below before reading on.

ACTIVITY

What can we do to control STD? look back at the problems you listed at and decide how you might overcome them.

____

____

____

____

Compare your notes with ours on the next page.

In order to reduce the spread of STD infection, we need to have strategies that are feasible, effective and affordable. These must include:

- early diagnosis and treatment of people with STD in order to reduce both i transmission to others and to minimize their consequences;
- educating patients (and the general public) on the dangers of unsafe sex and persuading them to use condoms and limit the number of sexual partners;
- treatment and education of sexual partners of people with STD; targeting vulnerable groups, such as sex workers.

Early, effective therapy

To achieve the goal of early treatment, all patients with STD need to be treated quickly and effectively at their first visit to a health facility. This will lead to the patient being both non-infectious and symptom-free, decreasing the risk of further transmission. In practical terms this means that STD services should be mode available at all health facilities.

For this to happen, all such facilities need adequate supplies of the necessary drugs. Equally, service providers need training in diagnosis and treatment of STD as well as all the other skills listed below.

Education and communication

Education is essential in order to encourage people to adopt safe sex practices, and to help those who are exposed to risk of infection by other people's behaviour. The aim of education is to ensure that treated patients remain free of infection and avoid transmitting STD further. It must therefore emphasis:

- the dangers of high-risk behaviour, including the risk of HIV;
- the range of low-risk behaviours, including non-penetrative sex and the use of condoms;
- the need for compliance with drug treatments - taking

a full course of the required drugs in the right dosage. Patients with STD often stop taking their medication when the symptoms decrease or go away. They need to appreciate the importance of continuing to take the drugs so the infection is fully cured.

Interviewing skills: To overcome people's resistance to changing behaviour or help them find ways to reduce their risk and the embarrassment connected with sex and STD, service providers must first win their patients' trust and confidence. To do this, they must be able to listen, question and advise each individual patient according to his or her circumstances.

Condom promotion: If used properly, condoms can prevent the spread of STD and HIV. All sexually active people should know how to use them. Service providers should be prepared to discuss and demonstrate condoms. Clearly, they must feel comfortable doing this.

Adopting a positive attitude: For many people STD carry a stigma: they are seen as shameful, even disgraceful and are often taboo subjects. To work effectively with STD patients, service providers must treat them with the respect they are due. In turn, this requires looking closely at our own attitudes to people with STD and HIV; all service providers must be open and positive.

Treating sexual partners

Known partners should be treated for the STD even if they have no symptoms themselves, so service providers must also encourage patients to inform partners. This is sometimes a difficult task for patients, one that they need to plan carefully, so a good relationship with the service provider is essential.

Targeting vulnerable groups

Both male and female commercial sex workers and their clients run the highest risk of becoming infected. The partners of these people are in turn at high risk of i infection .

Other vulnerable groups include those working away from home and those who use drugs. Many countries now have outreach service providers who work closely with vulnerable groups on risk reduction.

This first workbook has introduced you to the size and scope of the epidemic c sexually transmitted diseases. We have seen that, even given the limited statistics available, STD form a major burden on health services, individuals and national economies. The burden grows alarmingly.

At the same time, if you have seen the scope of the problem, you have also learned something about the essential characteristics of any effective management programme for STD: early diagnosis and treatment.

You should now be able to:

- identify how STD are transmitted and the key factors that influence transmission;
- appreciate the serious consequences and complications that can arise if they are untreated;
- explore the extent of STD and explain why it is so difficult to assess the trucburden;
- identify the two-way link between STD and the spread of HIV;
- explain why the control of STD is so difficult, and what must be done to achieve control.

To complete this first workbook, please turn to the Statistics Project.

F. STATISTICS PROJECT

Having learned about worldwide statistics on STD and HIV {their frequency and distribution), it would be helpful to find out more about the statistics available for your country, region or community.

This project is one that your trainer may ask you to work on with a study group.

If you can't join a study group, please discuss your findings with your collcagues and supervisor. Your supervisor should be able to help you access any available statistics or records.

There are three sets of activities: gathering information, interpreting the information, and drawing conclusions.

Gathering information

- Think about what sort of information would be useful to have about STD in your country or region, and why.
- Collect information that is available on STD and HIV for your country, region or community. Approach your local health service for any numbers they have on people seeking treatment for STD, and find out if any special surveys using laboratory tests have been done. (Your tutor or supervisor may be able to help you with statistics or other information.)
- Collect any estimates about STD or HIV in addition to, or perhaps in the absence of, statistics.

Interpreting the information

- According to the information you have gathered, who is most at risk of STD? Are particular groups more at risk than others?
- To what extent is this information useful, given your answers to question I above?

- How accurate can you consider the statistical (or estimates) to be?
- To what extent might the statistics ignore women, and why?

Drawing conclusions

- Make simple graphs or tables that show the information you have gathered.
- Make a list of conclusions that can be drown from the infirmation you have gathered.

G. ANSWERS

1. Well done if you spotted our introductory statement that "chancroid, chlamydia, gonorrhoea, syphilis and trichomoniasis may increase the risk of HIV transmission by 2 to 9 times".

The quotation from Population Reports provides findings for specific diseases, including:

	Increases risk of HIV transmission by:
Syphilis	3 - 9 times
Gonorrhoea	3 - 5 times
Chlamydia	3 - 5 times

The article also mentions genital herpes, reporting a doubled risk of transmission. Please note that this syndromic programme does not cover herpes, though you should always encourage patients with this virus to avoid sexual activity when a herpes sore is present.

Why do you think there is such a range in the available figures? In part, the range can result from the sheer problems of this type of research. Remember that we discussed these difficulties in this workbook.

2. The article suggests two possible reasons why non-ulcer causing STD increase the risk of transmitting HIV:
   (a) The presence of STD viruses or bacteria in the bloodstream locally stimulate the body's immune system to increase the number of white blood cells - which are both targets and sources of HIV.
   (b) Genital inflammation may cause microscopic cuts that allow HIV to enter the body.

3. HIV-infection may affect transmission of STD in two ways: by making an STD more resistant to treatment, and by making people more susceptible to STD

GLOSSARY

AIDS	Acquired Immune Deficiency Syndrome
Amniotic sac	Membranes that enclose amniotic fluid and the fetus in the womb
Antenatal	Period before giving birth
Cervix	Lower part of the uterus that protrudes into the vagina, often called the neck of the uterus
Chancroid	STD caused by the bacterium Haemophilus ducreyi; one of the causes of genital ulcers
Chlamydia	Infection with the bucterium Chlamydium trachomatis; one of the causes of vaginal and urethral discharge, and of discharging eyes in newborns
Complications	A secondary disease or condition that can arise if a disease is not treated
Congenital syphilis	Syphilis passed from the mother to the child during pregnancy
Conjunctivitis	Inflammation of the mucous membrane of the eyes and eyelids
Ectopic pregnancy	Pregnancy outside the uterus (usually in the *fallopian tubes*); a life-threatening condition, which can cause massive internal bleeding
Efficacy of transmission	Likelihood that the contact with an infective agent results in infection
Epidemiology	The study of the incidence, distribution and causes of a disease or infection in a population
Epididymis	Organ behind the testicle, which links the testicle with the spermatic cord
Epididymitis	Inflammation of the *epididymis*, usualy due to *gonorrhoea* or *chlumydia* infection
Fallopian tubes	The tubes which carry ova from the ovaries to the uterus
Flow-chart	A chart which shows the steps that need to be taken to perform a task
Genital lesions	Skin scars/injuries which break out in the genital region
Genital ulcer disease	The name for the *syndrome* where ulcers or sores are found in the genital region, usually caused by *syphilis* and *choncroid*
Gonorrhoea/gonorrhea	STD caused by the bacterium Neisseria *gonorrhoea*; common cause of urethral and vagina; discharge, and of discharging eyes in newborns
Gynaecological	Related to the female genital organs and their functions
Herpes	Common name for the Herpes *simplex virus* (HSV); a common cause of genital blisters and sores (also referred to in the flow-chart for genital ulcers as vesicular lesions)
HIV	Abbreviation for the Human Immunodeficiency virus which causes *AIDS*

Lymphogranuloma venereum	*STD* caused by a specific type of the bacterium *Chlamydium trachomatis*; one of the causes of genital ulcers and inguinal bubo
Natural history of an infection	The course of an infection if untreated (the natural history of different STD varies, for example, chancroid eventually heals on its own, whereas untreated syphilis may spread to other organs and lead to complications, even after many years)
Ophthalmia neonatorum	*Conjunctivitis* occurring in baby less than one month old, usually due to gonorrhoea or chlamydia infection
Pelvic inflammatory disease	Inflommation of the lower abdominal cavity involving the uterus, fallopian tubes and ovaries, usually due to *gonorrhoea* and *chlomydia* and/or anserobic bacteria
Perinatal	Around birth (shortly before or aher birth)
PlD	An abbreviation for pelvic inflammotory disease
Sexually transmitted diseases {STD)	Disease passed from one person to another through sexual intercourse
Sign(s}	A clinical problem you can see by examination (together with symptom(s) these make up a *syndrome*)
Susceptibility to infection	How much resistance the body has to infection (for example, little resistance would mean that patient was highly susceptible)
Symptomf(s)	A clinical problem which the patient complains of (together with sign(s) these make a *syndrome*)
Syndrome	Specific collection of *symptoms* and *signs*
Syndromic case management	Management of a patient on his/her STD syndrome rather than on the detection of a disease's specific causes
Syphilis	*STD* caused by the bacterium *Treponema pallidum*; one of the causes of genital ulcers
Trichomoniasis	*STD* caused by the micro-orgonism *Trichomonas* vaginalis; one of the causes of vaginal discharge
Urethra	Duct by which urine is discharged from the bladder
Urethral stricture	Narrowing of the urethra, caused by infection
Urethritis	Inflammation of the urethra, usually caused by gonorrhoea or chlamydia
Vertical transmission	Infection which passes down from the mother to the foetus or child

3

USING FLOW-CHARTS FOR SYNDROMIC MANAGEMENT

A. INTRODUCTION

This workbook introduces you to syndromic case management, how it works, and its advantages over the classic approaches to STD management.

Before starting this workbook, you should already have completed Workbook 1, so that you are aware of the scale of the STD epidemic, and the problems of reducing its transmission.

Other workbooks will develop your understanding of the flow-charts much further, by working through every step of each one in detail.

Your learning objectives

By the time you have completed this workbook and the activities that go with it, you will be able to:

- List a number of problems with the classic approaches to treating patients with STD;
- identify the main features of syndromic case management;
- outline various advantages that syndromic case management offers;
- List the steps in using flow-charts to treat patients;
- consider your further learning needs, which will depend on your responsibilities as a member of a health care team.

Resources

Please keep a copy of the seven flow-charts nearby when you are studying Section 3 of this workbook.

Remember: The quality of the syndromic case management approach will depend on you, the service provider.

B. APPROACHES TO DIAGNOSIS

Service providers generally use one of two approaches to STD diagnosis:

- *etiological diagnosis*: using laboratory tests to identify the causative agent;
- *clinical diagnosis*: using clinical experience tr identify symptoms, typical for a specific STD.

Etiological diagnosis is often regarded as the ideal approach in medicine. It enables service providers to make precise diagnoses and treat their patients with equal precision.

However, in the diagnosis and treatment of STD, both classical approaches present a number of problems.

Before reading on, please make some notes in answer to the question below:

What problems can you see with identifying a causative agent before offering treatment? (A tip: in Workbook 1 we said that early, effective therapy was essential to control the spread of STD. . .)

We have summarized the main problems of etiological and clinical diagnosis of STD opposite.

In fact, given the need to mount an effective challenge against STD, both approaches present problems.

Etiological diagnosis presents several significant problems:

1. Identifying the 20 or more STD causative agents requires both

skilled personnel and sometimes sophisticated laboratory equipment:

- gonococcal infections in men and trichomonas in women can be diagnosed through microscopy - but only if a microscope and trained microscopist are available;
- both gonococcal and chlamydial infections in women currently have to be diagnosed through sophisticated laboratory tests; culture techniques are technically demanding and are not always possible in primary health core settings;
- tests such as RPR and VDRL can be used to screen for syphilis, but they require serum or plasma;
- tests for herpes and other STD are even more complicated.

2. A large number of patients seek care for STD at the primary health care level, and at this level the required facilities and skills for etiological diagnosis are not available.
3. Etiological diagnosis is also expensive and time-consuming. There are inherent delays in reporting test results and hence in treatment of STD cases. Such delays can undermine a patient's confidence in the service provider-significant proportion of clients fail to attend clinics for follow-up treatment.

Some clinicians feel that, after examining a patient, it is easy to make a clinical diagnosis, such as gonococcal urethritis or chlamydial urethritis. However, even specialists sometimes misdiagnose STD when relying on their own clinical experience. Why? In many instances it is not possible to differentiate clinically between the various infections and, in addition, it is common for mixed infections to occur. A patient who has multiple infections needs to be treated for each of them. Failure to treat one infection may result in the development of serious complications as you saw in Workbook 1.

Summary

Even in a well-structured health system, etiological and clinical diagnosis are problematic. Etiological diagnosis is expensive and time-consuming; it requires special resources and delays treatment. With clinical diagnosis, it is easy to misdiagnose some STD and also to miss mixed infections.

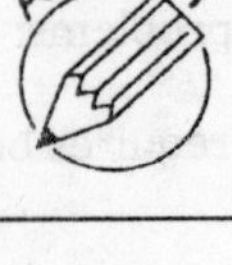

Do any of these problems with etiological and clinical diagnosis apply in your clinic or health centre? If so, which ones?

What might be the disadvantages of etiological diagnosis for your patients?

Please discuss these issues with colleagues if you have any doubts about the arguments we have used.

C. SYNDROMIC CASE MANAGEMENT

In this section we introduce you to a third approach to STD treatment - what is known as syndromic case management.

How does syndromic case management differ from the two approaches we discussed in Section 1 ? What are its main features and what benefits does it offer? We will try to answer these questions before moving on to section D, where re you will learn how the flow-charts work.

First let's explore the main features of syndromic case management. They are:

- classifying the main causative agents by the clinical syndromes to which they give rise;
- using flow-charts which help the service provider to identify causes of a given syndrome;
- treating the patient for all the important causes of the syndrome;
- ensuring that partners are treated, patients educated on treatment compliance and risk reduction, and condoms provided.

Over the next few pages, we'll explain these three features in more detail, and how they can help us attain the goal of rapid and effective treatment with STD.

For the moment, spend a few minutes noting down any questions or ideas you have about syndromic management.

____

____

____

____

____

____

Identifying the syndromes

Although STDs are caused by many different organisms, these organisms only give rise to a limited number of syndromes. A syndrome is simply a group of the symptoms of which a patient complains, and the signs observed during examination. This table explains the signs and symptoms for the main STD syndromes and their etiologies.

Syndrome	*Symptoms*	*Signs*	*Most common etiologies*
Vaginal discharge	Vaginal discharge Vaginal itching Dysuria (pain on urination} Pain during sexual relations	Vaginal discharge	VAGINITIS: - Trichomoniasis - Candidiasis CERVICITIS: - Gonorrhoea - Chlamydia
Urethral discharge	Urethral discharge Dysuria Frequent urination	Urethral discharge (if necessary ask patient to milk urethra)	Gonorrhoea Chlamydia
Genital ulcer	Genital sore	Genital ulcer Enlarged inguinal lymph nodes	Syphilis Chancroid Genital herpes
Lower abdominal pain	Lower abdominal pain and poin during sexual relations	Vaginal discharge Lower abdominal tenderness on palpation Temperature -38°	Gonorrhoea Chlamydia Mixed anaerobes
Scrotal swelling	Scrotal pain and swelling	Scrotal swelling	Gonorrhoea Chlamydia

Inguinal bubo	Painful enlarged inguinal lymph nodes	Swollen lymph nodes Fluctuation Abscesses or fistulae	LGV Chancroid
Neonatal conjunctivitis	Swollen eyelids Discharge Baby cannot open eyes	Oedema of the eyelids Purulent discharge	Gonorrhoea Chlamydia

The aim of syndromic management is to identify one of these seven syndromes and manage it accordingly.

It includes only those syndromes that are caused by organisms which both respond to treatment and lead to severe consequences if left untreated. Other STD, syndromes, such as vesicular lesions (herpes), genital warts and dysuria in women (painful passing urine), are not included among the seven syndromes in his programme.

Using syndromic flow-charts

Because the seven syndromes are easy to identify, it has been possible to devise 'flow-chart' for each one. Each flow-chart takes us carefully through the decisions and actions that we need to take, leading to guidance on the condition or conditions for which to treat the patient. Once trained, service providers will and the flow-charts easy to use, so it is possible for non-STD specialists at any health facility to manage STD cases.

If this is a key benefit of the flow-charts, what other benefits does it offer in turn?

- promptness of treatment, because STD services can be made available at any first-line health facility. Patients are thus treated at their first visit;
- wider access to treatment, because treatment is availsble at more heolth centres, so resching for more of the population;
- opportunities for introducing preventive and promotive measures such as education and distribution of condoms.

Treatment for all the causative agents

While a clinical or etiological diagnosis tries to identify just one causative agent, syndromic diagnosis includes immediate treatment for all the most important causative agents.

This means that- if all the necessary drugs are available- syndromic treatment will quickly render the patient non-infectious. As we discussed in Workbook 1, mixed infections occur quite often, so the costs of over-treatment can be balanced against the cost of failing to treat people for mixed or symptom-free infections.

Let's tske an example to show how syndromic disgnosis and treatment works.

A patient complains of having noticed a discharge from the penis. Upon examination, you notice a discharge from the urethra. The sign and symptom together suggest urethral discharge syndrome. Urethral discharge syndrome is caused, most of the time, by gonorrhoea and chlamydial infection, so any treatment advised should be effective against both these causes.

There are other causes of urethral discharge syndrome, such as infection with Ureaplasma urealyticum and Trichomonas vaginalis. Should the patient be treated for these causes as well? Not necessarily, because both are less common and do not lead to complications. Their treatment syndromically is not urgent. However, both gonorrhoea and chlamydial infection are common; not only can they cause complications, but they can facilitate the transmission and acquisition of HIV. So it is essential that we treat the patient for both of these.

As this example shows, we can use syndromic management to identify the most likely causes of a patient's symptoms and signs, and treat the patient for those that have serious complications or sequelae.

Here is another example that you might like to work on.

A young woman complains of a sore and upon examination you notice an ulcer on the outer labia. This indicates the syndrome of genital ulcer.

There are two main causes of genital ulcer: chancroid and syphilis. How should you manage this young woman's treatment? There are a number of possibilities.

QUESTION

1. *How would you manage the treatment for genital ulcer? Tick the option you think best out of the list below:*

   (a) *Treat the patient for one cause only, and ask the patient to return if the sore doesn't get better, so you can then treat for the second cause.*

   (b) *Teat the patient for both conditions immediately.*

   (c) *Refer the patient for an etiological giagnosis.*

When discussing syndromic diagnosis with any group of people, we find that they tend to raise similar criticisms. Below is a summary of their criticisms. Please note down whether you agree or disagree with each one, and why, and then read our comments over the page.

'The syndromic approsch isn't scientific.'

'Syndromic diognosis is far too simple for a physicion to us–it can even be used by nurses.'

'The syndromic approach fails to make use of a service provider's clinical skills and experience.'

'It would be better to treat the patient first for the most common cause and then, if the symptoms don't improve, treat for a second cause.'

The syndromic approach results in a waste of drugs because patients are being over-treated.'

'Good, simple laboratory tests such as Gram stain should be included in STD diagnosis.'

Responding to criticisms of the syndromic approach

Below we have tried to answer the main criticisms made against the syndromic approsch. Many of our comments touch on points we have already raised, both in Workbook 1 and so far in this workbook, so the activity was partly intended to help you review the arguments - though it adds some interesting detsils:

'The syndromic approach isn't scientific'.

On the contrary, it is based on a wide range of epidemiological studies over the industrialized and developing world. A number of validation studies compared syndromic and loboratory diagnosis to assess the accuracy of syndromic diagnosis. They found syndromic diagnosis to be similar, and hence accurute. As a result, syndromic diagnosis of STD has been taken up even in hospitals in both Amsterdam and London.

'Syndromic diagnosis is far too simple for a physician to use - it can even be used by nurses'.

Simplicity does not prevent physicians from using other tools including thermometer or stethoscope! And surely it is an advantage that other service providers can use a syndromic approach to diagnosis? For example, in the Netherlands, nurses have been using syndromic diagnosis to treat STD patients for a number of years. Simplified diagnosis and treatment also allows health workers more time to provide education and counselling.

'The syndromic approach fails to make use of a service provider's clinical skills and experience.'

Many clinicians rely too much on their own clinical judgement. They don't want to face the fact that they can make a clinical diagnosis in only 50% of STD cases. They also miss all the mixed infections.

'It would be better to treat the patient first for the most common cause and then if the symptoms don't improve, treat for a second cause.'

We hope you spotted this one! It is exactly the point we tried to make in our answer to question 1. Patients who are not cured by the first treatment may not return to the hesith centre and may even seek treatment elsewhere. They may also become asymptomatic in the untreated STD and further spread the infection.

'The syndromic approach results in a waste of drugs, because patients are being over-treated'.

In fact studies have shown that the syndromic approach is the most cost-effective in the long run. Why? Because of the comparatively large costs of technology, skills and infrastructure of an etiological approach, and the long-term costs of failed treatment of, and clinical diagnosis based on experience only.

'Good, simple laboratory tests such as Gram stain should be included in STD dragnosis.'

No! Patients have to wait for the results and may not return for treatment. They also stay infectious and complications can occur. Gram stain is only justified when microscopy is already available, rapidly performed and accurate.

Summary

In this section we have introduced you to the syndromic approach to STD case management. You have learned why and how the syndromic approach is so effective. Indeed it is the only approach that meets the main need to control the spread of STD: early, effective treatment at a patient's first visit to a health facility.

We also identified the three main features of the syndromic approach:

- classifying the main causative agents by the clinical syndromes to which they give rise;
- using flow-charts which help the first-line service provider to identify causes of a given syndrome;
- prompt treatment for all the important causes of the syndrome;
- ensuring that partners are treated, patients educated on trestment compliance and risk reductions, and condoms promoted.

Now we need to add all the other features essential for comprehensive STD case management, which we mentioned at the end of Workbook 1:

- availability of the appropriate drugs;
- education on how to reduce the risk of reinfection and complying with treatment;
- provision and promotion of condoms;
- treatment of the patient's sexual partners.

In the next section we'll introduce you to the flow-charts we have talked so much about!

> *Remember: rapid and effective treatment of people with STD is the best way to interrupt the cycle of transmission. For the purpose of STD control, syndromic management is the best approach devised.*

D. USING THE FLOW-CHARTS

This section introduces you to the STD case management flow-charts. They are essential tools in the syndromic approach because they enable non-specialists in STD to diagnose and treat STD patients.

The section explains what a flow-chart is, and how the flow-charts for syndromic case management work. It also gives you a number of exercises which will help you to get used to the flow-charts.

You will also have the opportunity to note questions and problems as you work through the section. Please discuss these with your colleagues if the section does not provide ready answers!

For more practical guidance on using each of the flow-charts, you will find Workbook 4 very helpful. It also provides guidance on the recommended drug treatments.

Please have a copy of all the flow-charts with you when you study this section.

What is a flow-chart?

A flow-chart is a decision and action tree. It guides the reader through a series of decisions and actions that need to be made. Each decision or action is enclosed in a box, with one or two routes leading out of it to another box, with another decision or action.

Upon learning a patient's symptoms, the service provider turns to the relevant flow-chart and works through the decisions and actions it suggests.

Each flow-chart is made up of a series of three steps. These are:

- the clinical problem (when using the flow-charts, the pstient's presenting symptom);
- the decision that needs to be taken;
- the action that needs to be carried out.

If you have already glanced at the flow-charts, like many people you might feel rather awed by their complexity - especially if you haven't seen a flow-chart before. Please don't worry: they are not difficult to use, as you will very soon see.

Here is an example. (See next page).

To use a flow-chart, simply start at the clinical problem box and work step by step through the decision tree until you arrive at an action box at the end of a branch.

Here is the flow-chart for urethral discharge. (See next page).

This flow-chart is more complicated than the one for enlarged inguinal lymph nodes because it has two decision boxes, but you will find that it is just as easy to use. Simply remember that you must work through it step by step. Never jump or skip over any steps.

The flow-chart has two decision boxes and four action boxes. One action box is about examining the patient and one refers you to another flow-chart.

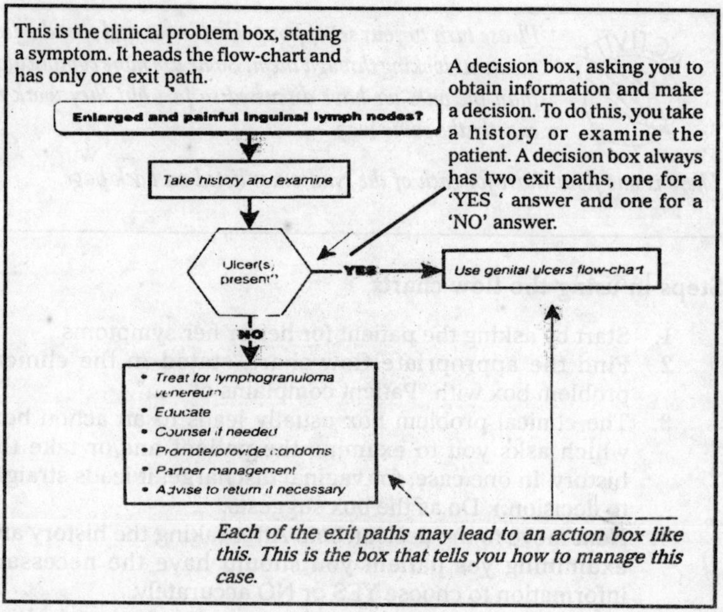
This is the clinical problem box, stating a symptom. It heads the flow-chart and has only one exit path.
A decision box, asking you to obtain information and make a decision. To do this, you take a history or examine the patient. A decision box always has two exit paths, one for a 'YES ' answer and one for a 'NO' answer.
Enlarged and painful inguinal lymph nodes?
Take history and examine
Ulcer(s) present?
YES
Use genital ulcers flow-chart
NO
• Treat for lymphogranuloma venereum
• Educate
• Counsel if needed
• Promote/provide condoms
• Partner management
• Advise to return if necessary
Each of the exit paths may lead to an action box like this. This is the box that tells you how to manage this case.

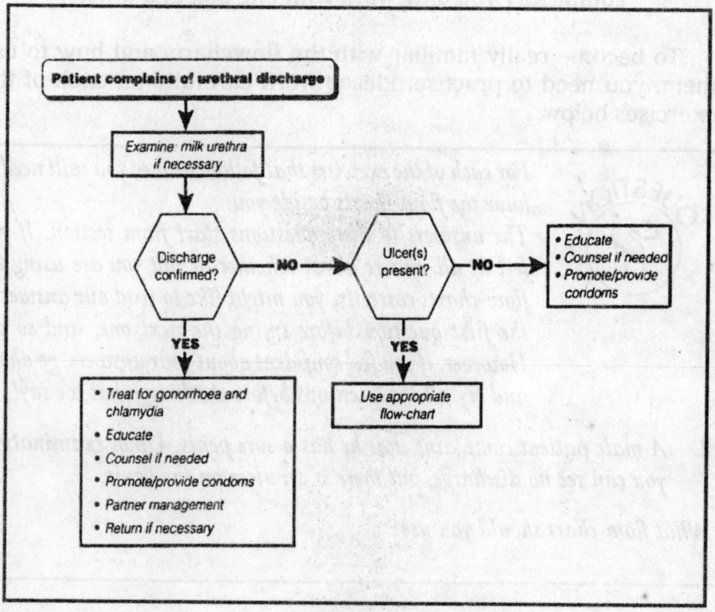
Patient complains of urethral discharge
Examine: milk urethra if necessary
Discharge confirmed?
NO
Ulcer(s) present?
NO
• Educate
• Counsel if needed
• Promote/provide condoms
YES
• Treat for gonorrhoea and chlamydia
• Educate
• Counsel if needed
• Promote/provide condoms
• Partner management
• Return if necessary
YES
Use appropriate flow-chart

Please turn to your set of flow-charts now and spend a few moments looking through them. Some are more complicated than the ones we have discussed so far, but they work in exactly the same way.

There is one flow-chart for each of the syndromes listed on back page.

Steps in using the flow-charts

1. Start by asking the patient for her or her symptoms.
2. Find the appropriate flow-chart, stated in the clinical problem box with "Patient complains of ......".
3. The clinical problem box usually leads to an action box, which asks you to examine the patient and/or take the history. In one case, for vaginal discharge, it leads straight to decision.) Do as the box suggests.
4. Next move to the decison box. After taking the history and examining yes patient you should have the necessary information to choose YES or NO accurately.
5. Depending on your choice, there may be further decision boxes and action boxes. Don't be confused by its apparent complexity you only work with one box at a time.

To become really familiar with the flowcharts and how to use them, you need to practise. Please work carefully on each of the exercises below.

For each of the exercises that follow below, you will need to have the flow-charts beside you.
The answers to these questions start from section. If you feel at all unsure about whether or not you are using the flow-charts correctly, you might like to read our answer to the first question before trying the next one, and so on. However, if you feel confident about your answers, go ahead and try all the questions before checking what we say!

2. *A male patient complains that he has a sore penis. Upon examination, you can see no discharge, but there is an ulcer on the penis.*

What flow-chart should you use?

For what action do you need to take?

3. *A young woman complains of a pain in her stomach, low down. You take her history and examine her. She tells you that her periods are normal and she has never been pregnant. She has no rebound tenderness but clearly feels pain when you palpate her abdomen.*

What flow-chart should you use?

For what action do you need to take?

A week later, the same woman returns. She tells you that she feels no better, though she took all the tablets you gave her as you suggested. Upon examination, you discover that she has a temperature of 38.2° C.

What action do you now take?

4. *A middle-aged man tells you that he has felt pain in his groin for a week or so. Upon examination, you confirm that he has a painful fluctuating mass in the right groin. The patient winces, although you have been very gentle in your examination. There are no ulcers on his penis.*

What flow-chart should you use?

For what do you treat him?

5. *A woman attending clinic with her four-day-old baby asks you to look at his eyes. You notice that his eyelids are swollen and there is a purulent discharge in both eyes.*

What flow-chart should you use?

For what do you treat the child?

Who else do you treat, and for what?

The mother returns with the child three days later. There is no improvement in the discharge. What do you do now?

After a few more days the mother and child return again. The child's eyes are less swollen. What do you do now?

6. *A young man complains of a swollen scrotum. An examination confirms the swelling but the testis is not rotated or elevated and there is no history of trauma.*

What flow-chart should you use?

For what do you treat him?

7. *A young man tells you shyly that he has a discharge from his penis. You ask him to milk his urethra; upon his doing so, you confirm that there is a slight discharge. There are no other lesions or ulcers.*

What flow-chart do you use?

For what do you treat the patient?

How did you do with the five questions? If you got most of them right and can understand any mistakes you made, you can safely say that you understand the basic way to use the flow-charts to treat patients with STD. Other workbooks will provide full details on diagnosis and treatment, including what 'risk assessment' is, and what drugs are recommended by WHO.

How do these flow-charts help?

There are a number of advantages in using these flow-charts to treat STD:

- you and your colleagues are able to offer STD case management for all the patients you see as part of your everyday work at the health facility;
- you do not need specialist equipment and there is usually

no need to refer patients to more specialized clinics or centres;

- the flow-charts suggest clear decisions and actions to follow on a step-by-step basis;
- once your health facility has the necessary drugs and all the service providers to be involved have been trained, the flow-charts offer everyone the chance to follow clear, shared, guidelines.

At this point in learning about syndromic case management of STD, people tend to have lots of questions. You may be one of them, so please give some time to this activity.

Having almost completed Workbook 2, note down:

- *any questions that you still have about syndromic case management of STD;*
- *any problems you anticipate in implementing syndromic case management at your health centre;*
- *any possible benefits that syndromic case management will bring.*

E. REVIEW

In this workbook, we have introduced you to syndromic case management of people with STD. You should now be able to:

- outline a number of problems with classical approaches to the diagnosis and treatment of STD;
- identify the three main features of syndromic case management of STD;

- respond to the most often-heard criticisms of syndromic case management.
- List four additional features that are essential to comprehensive case management:
  — availability of the appropriate drugs;
  — education on:
    treatment compliance;
    risk reduction;
  — promotion and provision of condoms;
  — treatment of sexual partners.

You have also learned the basic steps in using the flow-charts as part of syndromic case management, and explored their advantages as well as any problems you anticipate.

It is essential to reduce the spread of STD and the cycle of transmission and re-infection. Syndromic case management can help you do this. This course has been designed to help you provide the best service possible.

Please explore syndromic case management further with your colleagues or supervisor. On the next page you'll find some tips to help you become more familiar with the flow-charts and syndromic case management.

Workbook 3 will help you to develop the skills necessary for the first step in syndromic case management: taking the patient's history and examining the patient.

Best wishes with the rest of your learning!

F. ACTION PLAN

Below are some tips for your self-development as you continue to study.

1. Keep the flow-charts to hand at all times. If possible, place them on a desk or, better, on a wall, where you can see them easily. (Check: a wall-chart or pocket version may be available.)
2. Glance back page and the points you wrote down. Arrange to discuss those questions with colleagues or your tutor or supervisor.
3. If you have not already done so, plan the rest of your learning as we described in the Programme Introduction. For example, you may or may not be personally involved in all six responsibilities in STD case management; if you are at all unsure, discuss with your manager what your responsibilities will be.
4. If one of your colleagues is already using the syndromic

approach, try to arrange to observe him or her. You might pick up valuable tips to make your own learning easier. (But please remember: always ask the patient for his or her permission to observe, and respect the patient's right to privacy at all times.)

G. ANSWERS

1. Well done if you chose b) as the answer to this question. Clinically, it is not possible to distinguish the cause of a genital ulcer with any accuracy, so the safest option is prompt treatment for both causative agents, leaving the patient no longer infectious.

   Option a) presents problems typical of a clinical apprasch to diagnosis an treatment. If the patient is not cured by the first treatment, she may spread the infection. There is also a further risk that the patient might seek treatment elsewhere and managed inadequately.
   If you ticked c): '*Refer the patient for an etiological diagnosis*', remember that, in the first section, we stressed the many problems that can arise from a delay in treatment- even supposing the necessary tests are available locally.

2. A male patient complains that he has a sore penis. Upon examination, you can see no discharge, but there is an ulcer on the penis.

The correct flow-chart to use for this patient is the one for genital ulcers.

Well done if you wrote that you should treat the patient for syphilis and chancroid.

3. A young woman complains of a pain in her stomach, low down. You take her history and examine her. She tells you that her periods are normal and she has never been pregnant. She has no rebound tenderness but clearly feels pain when you palpate her abdomen.

Well done if you decided to use the flow-chart for lower abdominal pain.

The flow-chart lists five actions that you need to take:

- treat for PID;
- educate the patient;
- counsel if needed;
- promote/provide condoms;
- partner management.

When, a week later, she tells you that she feels no better, and you discover that she has a high temperature, you need to refer her for further treatment.

4. A middle-aged man tells you that he has felt pain in his groin for a week or so. Upon examination, you confirm that he has an inguinal bubo. The patient winces, although you have been very gentle in your examination. There are no ulcers on his penis.

You are quite right if you wrote that the flow-chart to use is the one for inguinal bubo, and that you treat him for lymphogranuloma venereum.

5. A woman attending clinic with her four-day-old baby asks you to look at his eyes. You notice that his eyelids are swollen and there is a purulent discharge in both eyes.

For these signs use the flow-chart for neonatal conjunctivitis, which tells you to treat the child for gonorrhoea.

Well done if you noticed that you need also to treat both the mother and her partner or partners. While the child is treated for just gonorrhoea, the adults must be treated for gonorrhoea and chlamydia.

If there is no improvement in the discharge after three days, treat the child for chlamydia, asking the mother to return in one week's time.

When they return for the second time, and you find the eyes are responding to treatment, all you do is reassure the mother that the treatment is working, and urge her to continue with it.

6. A young man complains of a swollen scrotum. An examination confirms the swelling but the testis is not rotated or elevated and there is no history of trauma.

The right flow-chart to use for this patient is the one on scrotal swelling.

Well done if you arrived at the action box that tells you to treat him for gonorrhoea and chlamydia.

7. A young man tells you shyly that he has a discharge from his penis. You ask him to milk his urethra; upon his doing so, you confirm that there is a slight discharge. There are no other lesions or ulcers.

The correct flow-chart for this syndrome is the one for urethral discharge. You should treat this patient for both gonorrhoea and chlamydia.

GLOSSARY

Action box	The rectangular box on a flow-chart that tells you to do something, for example, take history, treat or educate
Anaerobic bacteria	One of the causes of PID, bacteria (usually

	Bacteriodes) that grow without air or need an oxygen-free environment to live
Asymptomatic	Free of *symptoms* (ie where the patient does not complain of any symptoms)
Candida albicans	Scientific name for the yeastlike fungus (also known as 'thrush') that is one of the causes of *vaginitis*
Candidiasis	A common name for *Candida olbiscans*, one of the causes of *vaginitis*
Cervicitis	Inflammation of the cervix, usually caused by *gonorrhoea or chlamydia*
Chancroid	STD caused by the bacterium *Haemophilus ducreyi*
Chlamydia	STD caused by the bacterium *Chlamydia trachomatis*
Chlamydial	Caused by chlamydia, as in chlamydial urethritis
Clinical diagnosis	Using clinical experience to identify an *STD*
Clinical problem box	The highlighted box on a flow-chart that states the typical symptom(s) of a particular syndrome
Comprehensive case	Treatment of *STD* that also includes education, management counselling and *partner management*
Culture techniques	Growing micro-organisms in sterile conditions to assist their identification
Decision box	The six-sided box on a flow-chart that asks you to obtain information and make a decision
Dysuria	Pain on urination
Etiologic/etiological	Using laboratory tests or microscopy to identify a causative agent
Etiologies	Causative agents
Fistulae	Abnormal passage between a hollow organ and the skin surface
Fluctuation	Movement of fluid such as pus within a bubo
	Gardnerella vaginalis One of the causes of vaginitis
Genital ulcer syndrome	The name for the syndrome where a patient presents with an ulcer or sore in the genital region, usually caused by *syphilis* or *chancroid*
Gonococcal	Caused by *gonorrhoea*, as in gonococcal urethritis
Gonorrhoea/gonorrhea	*STD* caused by the bacterium Neisseria gonorrhoea
Gram stain	Laboratory technique used to identify bacteria
Herpes	*STD* caused by Herpes simplex virus /HSV)
HIV	Abbreviation for 'human immunodeficiency virus' the causative agent of AIDS
Inguinal bubo{es}	The name of the *syndrome* where patients present with painful swellings) of the Iymph nodes in the groin, usually caused by *chlamydia*
Inguinal Iymph nodes	Lymph nodes in the groin
Lower abdominal pain	The name of the syndrome where women present with pain in the lower abdomen, usually- but not always - caused by pelvic inflammatory disease
Neonatal conjunctivitis	*Purulent conjunctivitis* occurring in a baby less than one month old, another name for *ophtholmia neonotorum*
Oedema	Swelling
Palpate/palpation	To examine by touch

Partner management	Contacting, treating and educating all the sexual partners of a patient treated for STD
Pelvic inflammatory disease	A general term covering the infections of the female genital tract that often prompt a patient to present with the syndrome of lower abdominal pain, usually caused by gonorrhoea, chlamydia or anaerobic bacteria
PID	An abbreviation for *pelvic inflammatory disease*
Plasma	Colourless fluid that is part of blood, lymph or milk
Purulent	Discharging pus
Rebound tenderness	One of the signs of peritonitis or an intra-*abdominal abscess* which you would look for during an examination for the syndrome lower abdominal *pain*. The patient will feel severe pain when you press down slowly and gently on a tender area and then suddenly release the pressure. Along with guording it is usually a sign of potentially serious conditions)
RPR	An abbreviation for 'rapid plasma reagin' one of the laboratory tests used to identify *syphilis* (see also *VRDL*)
Scrotal swelling	The name for the *syndrome* where men present with swollen, hot and painful *testis/testes* usually - but not always - caused by *gonorrhoea* or *chlamydia*
Serum	The amber coloured liquid that separates from blood after coagulation
Signs	A clinical problem you can see (contrast with symptoms)
STD	An abbreviation for sexually transmitted disease(s)
Symptom	A clinical problem that the patient complains of, together with signs making up a syndrome
	A collection of symptoms and signs
Syndromic case management	A method of treating all the causative agents of a *syndrome*
Syphilis	*STD* caused by the bacterium *Treponema pallidum*
Testis/testes	The medical name for a testicle or testicles
Trauma	Any physical wound or injury, sometimes also used to describe the shock following a wound or injury
Trichomonas vaginalis	The scientific name for the bacterium which causes the *STD trichomoniasis*
Trichomoniasis	*STD* caused by the bacterium *Trichomonas vaginalis*
Ureaplasma urealyticum	The scientific name for the bacterium that can be one of the causative agents for *vaginal discharge syndrome*
Urethra	The duct by which urine is discharged from the bladder (see also *urethritis*)
Urethral discharge	The name of the syndrome where men present with a discharge from their penis, usually caused by *gonorrhoea or chlamydia*
Urethritis	Inflammation of the urethra, caused by *gonorrhoea or chlamydia*

Vaginal discharge — The name of the *syndrome* where women present with a vaginal discharge which can be caused by *vaginitis* or *cervicitis*

Vaginitis — Inflammation of the vagina, caused by *trichomoniasis* or *candidiasis*

Vesicular lesions — Small blister-like sores that are a characteristic sign at *herpes*

VRDL — An abbreviation for 'Venereal Disease Research Laboratory' which is the name of a test used to identify *syphilis* (see also *RPR*)

4

HISTORY-TAKING AND EXAMINATION

A. INTRODUCTION

This workbook is about two very important skills in syndromic diagnosis: history-taking and examination. It will help you to take a useful history from a patient and also to carry out a physical examination.

By now you know that, in order to manage patients with any kind of illness, we need to know what symptoms and signs they have. We learn their symptoms by taking a history and identify any signs by examining them. This enables us to decide which flow-chart to use - and so treat the patient appropriately.

It is important to understand from the start that, even if you have a good deal of experience in interviewing patients, interviewing someone with symptoms of an STD is unique. Why is it unique? Because these symptoms occur in the genital area, causing the patient some degree of embarrassment: he or she may withhold such sensitive information or have difficulty answering your questions accurately.

So, in addition to questioning the patient effectively, you need quickly to win their trust and confidence if you are to take an accurate history in the short time you have available.

This workbook will, therefore, help you to refine your skills in communication and examination .

Take history → *Examine the patient*

In order to use any flow-chart effectively, you must first acquire or refine your interviewing and examination skills.

Your learning objectives

By the end of this workbook you should be able to take a history from a patient who has STD and carry out a physical examination. You will be able to:

- help the patient feel at ease;
- question the patient effectively, so that you gain their confidence and obtain a complete history;
- handle the patient's emotions appropriately;
- identify the information you need to collect to help you make a syndromic diagnosis;
- examine a patient with STD.

Your action plan

History-taking and examination cannot be learned simply by studying a workbook. To reach an appropriate standard in these skills - and to feel confident in what you are doing - you need to practise the skills.

If you are studying on your own, the action plans in the workbook will help you to do this. They ask you to practise with one or two other service providers, taking turns to be the patient and interviewer. When interviewing and examining a patient, you may have as little as ten minutes, or even five - so you need both experience and confidence!

B. THE PRINCIPLES OF EFFECTIVE COMMUNICATION

History-taking and examination are only two of the steps that take place in a typical encounter between service provider and patient with STD. The other steps include diagnosis and treatment, education and counselling and partner management - we will explore each of these steps in later workbooks. However, right now we want to stress that the skills you will refine with this workbook are ones you will need during most of the encounter.

By the end of this section you will be better able to:

- identify the aims of history-taking and examination;
- explain why it is so important to communicate effectively with an STD patient;
- offer patients privacy and confidentiality;
- identify the essential features of positive non-verbal communication.

First, let's establish the aims of this part of the interview. In common with any medical interview, one aim is to make a diagnosis which is both accurate, based on the history and examination, and efficient, given the time available for your task.

In STD case management, there are two further aims:

- to establish the patient's *risk* of contracting or transmitting STD;
- to find out about partners who may have been infected.

To explore the issues this raises, please answer the questions on the next page, and then read our comments.

1. *Given that some people may already be nervous about attending a health centre, consider how they might feel if they had any symptoms in their genital area - for example, an ulcer or unusual discharge. It might help to think how YOU would feel if you were to present such symptoms. As honestly as you can, note down those feelings.*

2. *As a service provider faced with interviewing someone with an STD, how do you feel about asking very personal questions - such as about their symptoms and their sexual partners? Imagine a person older than you or a member of the opposite sex and, once again, make notes as honestly as you can.*

So far, we have illustrated some of the difficulties connected with interviewing a patient with STD symptoms. We have also suggested three aims for these steps in the interview.

To meet these aims, your primary task is to establish a good *rapport* with the patient. Working with STD patients, the successful service provider will be positive, friendly and able to *empathise* with the patient (identify with their feelings).

Establishing a good rapport with the patient

How can we can establish a good rapport with a patient? This is where our communication skills come in:

- our verbal skills: the way we talk to the patient and ask questions;
- our non-verbal skills: how we behave towards the patient.

We will explore verbal skills in the next section and concentrate now on the nonverbal skills. Please read the case study below, and then answer questions 3 and 4 that follow it.

Amina is a nurse at a local clinic. She has had a very busy morning. She is still writing notes for a colleague who is standing beside her table, when the next patient enters the room. Amina glances briefly at the patient and says "Just a moment". The young woman shuffles her feet and stares at the floor. When Amina finishes writing, she leans back in her chair, sighs and puts her hands on the desk. Then she looks up sharply at the patient and asks: "What's your problem?".

The patient stands still, looking at the ground and shuffling her feet nervously. Amina's colleague picks up her note and leaves the room.

Amina repeats her question impatiently. "Well miss" responds the young woman, "I er. . . I haven 't been feeling very well. . . er.. . it's my tummy, it's..

"Goodness me! I haven't got all day!" says Amina. The patient begins to cry,

3. *If YOU were Amina 's patient, how would you FEEL?*

4. *What is WRONG with the way this young woman has been treated? Note down everything you can think of.*

The service provider in our case study made a lot of mistakes, so what should we do to establish rapport? Obviously, the first step should be to greet the patient in an appropriately friendly manner and introduce yourself, as you would like anyone else to do to you.

The key to effective non-verbal behaviour is to treat the patient with respect, and give him or her your full attention:

- *provide the patient with privacy.* Clearly, privacy and confidentiality are essential, so the interview must take place somewhere quiet where you won't be disturbed;
- *establish eye contact with the patient.* Look directly at him or her; in this way you can watch for key feelings that will help you to respond appropriately. The only time to avoid eye contact is when a patient seems very angry, since a direct gaze could be interpreted as aggressive. (In some parts of the world looking at people directly in the eye is considered rude and should be avoided.)
- *Listen carefully to what the patient says.* Show that you are listening by leaning forward slightly towards the patient; nod your head or comment occasionally to encourage them. Don't fidget or write while the patient is talking, and don't interrupt him or her;
- *sit if the patient is sitting* and stand when the patient stands; stay as close to the patient as is culturally acceptable - much better to be beside a table or desk than behind one!

These four points are very simple and they can make the difference between gaining or losing the patient's trust or confidence. Can any of us be sure that we practise such behaviours with all patients?

Summary

In this section we have explored the non-verbal aspects of good communication, suggesting four key behoviours that help the service provider establish rapport.

We have also stressed that any service provider who hopes to gain the patient's trust must use appropriate non-verbal language-behaving attentively and showing respect for the patient.

Next, you will learn or review a number of questioning techniques that will help you achieve your objectives in taking a history.

To complete this first section on the principles of good communication, please work on the activities on the next page.

Ensuring privacy and confidentiality

(a) *Consider your own working environment: to what extent can you interview patients in privacy?*

(b) *If you foresee difficulties in providing somewhere private for the interview, please discuss this important issue with your colleagues or supervisor.*

Refining your non-verbal skills

Luckily, non-verbal behaviour takes place in every face-to-face communication between two or more people so, if you would like to develop or refine your interpersonal skills and awareness, you will have ample opportunity! Here are some suggestions.

(a) *Often, non-verbal and verbal behaviour conflict, as when a colleague who LOOKS tired or harassed tells you that he or she "is fine". Pay close attention to other people's non-verbal behaviour over the next few days. How often does it confirm what someone is saying? How often does it tell you something extra or different about the person's feelings?*

(b) *Because non-verbal behaviour is often unconscious, we are not always aware of the messages that we are giving to other people. It's important to develop your own awareness: when you are talking to colleagues or friends, check your hands, facial expression and body posture. What are they telling other people about your own feelings?*

(c) *With a group of colleagues, discuss non-verbal communication questions like these:*

- *How do we convey feelings such as tiredness, frustration, impatience, anger, joy and depression, for example?*
- *What examples can each of you share about observing non-verbal behaviour? Does anyone have a good example of non-verbal behaviour conflicting or confirming what someone says?*

C. VERBAL SKILLS IN HISTORY-TAKING

Having looked at ways in which we can effectively communicate non-verbally, in this section we focus on how we question the patient and relieve their anxiety. We will also explore some characteristics of good interviewing practice which draw together both non-verbal and spoken skills.

This section will enable you to:

- use 'open' and 'closed' questions effectively during the interview;
- identify a number of extra verbal skills that will help you gather information effectively and to deal with the patient's emotions;
- summarise the characteristics of good interviewing practice.

Asking questions

As Section D will illustrate, you need to gather a lot of information from each STD patient: questions not only about their symptoms and their medical history, but about their sexual history also. You need to gather this information in a short time, so how can you best do this?

To draw on your own experience, please try these questions.

QUESTION

5. *There is something wrong with each of the six questions below and on the next page. Consider how you would feel answering each one, and then note how you think it could be improved.*

(a) (At the start of the interview) "Name?"

(b) "Tell me your medical history."

(c) "How many sexual partners have you had, when and who are they?"

(d) *"Have you had sex with people other than your husband?"*

___

___

___

(e) *"The symptoms only recur during your periods, don't they?"*

___

___

___

(f) *"Are your menses normal?"*

___

___

___

Exercise 5 raised some useful general tips for questioning patients:

- always phrase your questions politely and respectfully, however busy or rushed you may be;
- use words that the patient understands. Avoid using medical terms they may not understand;
- make your questions specific, so that the patient knows exactly how to answer you;
- ask one question at a time: double questions confuse;
- keep your questions free of moral judgements;
- avoid 'leading' questions that ask the patient to agree with you: let people answer in their own words;
- ask the patient's permission to question them about their STD or their sexual behoviour.

Open and closed questions

When talking to anyone, there are broadly two sorts of questions we can ask: closed questions and open questions.

Closed questions are ones that ask a patient to answer in one word or a short phrase, often with "yes" or "no":

"Is the swelling painful?"
"Is your period late?"
"Do you have a regular partner?"
"What is your age?"

"Where do you live?"
Open questions enable the patient to give a longer reply:

"What is troubling you?"
"What kind of medicines are you taking at the moment?"

Open-ended questions allow the patient to explain what's wrong or how they feel in their own words, and to tell you everything they think is important. Closed questions, on the other hand, ask the patient to answer a precise question in the service provider's words.

How can we best use the two types of question? Patients often have trouble revealing information about their own sexuality, so open questions will help them to be more comfortable when you begin the questions. Generally, you will also gather much more information from one open question than you can from a closed one.

There is another difficulty with using closed questions early in the interview - this is the danger of missing important information. Contrast this example of closed questions with the example that follows it:

Example 1

Patient:	I have a pain in my tummy.
Service provider:	I'm sorry to hear that. Where is the pain?
Patient:	Here.
Service provider:	Is it the pain constant?
Patient:	No.
Service provider:	Does it feel tender?
Patient:	Yes.
Service provider:	When did the pain begin?
Patient:	Last week.

Example 2

Patient:	I have a pain in my tummy.
Service provider:	I'm sorry to hear that. Tell me about this pain.
Patient:	Well, it started a week ago. At first I just felt tende down here, but sometimes it begins to hurt a lot. It hurts when I sit down or stand up - it isn't like my monthly pain at all.
Service provider:	What else is troubling you?
Patient:	Well, there is one other thing. There's a funny kind of water that I don 't usually get. It doesn 't hurt but it's embarrassing.

In the second example, the service provider has gathered more information by using open questions: "Tell me about this pain" and

"What else is troubling you?". Experts in interviewing STD patients suggests that we need to ask "Anything else?" several times, because some patients are so embarrassed about STD symptoms that they present first with other, quite unrelated symptoms - such as a headache!

Once you are sure that you have a complete understanding of the patient's problem as he or she sees it, closed questions may be very helpful to draw out specific details that you need to know.

It may help to think of open and closed questions as a triangle:

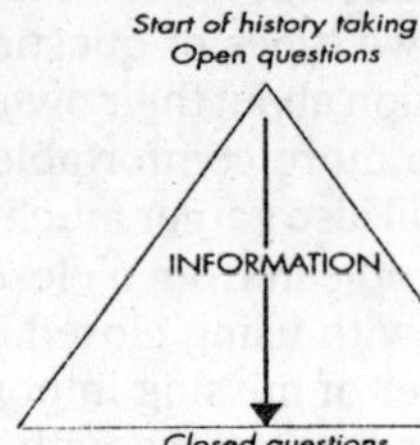

If you are learning about open and closed questions for the first time, the questions that follow will help you to check your understanding of them.

QUESTION

6. Which of these are open questions?

	Open? √
Do you have a discharge?	
Are you married?	
What is troubling you?	
Is it painful?	
Did you use a condom last time you had sex?	
Is the discharge milky or clear?	
What does the pain feel like? Tell me about your periods.	

7. *Below are four statements. Tick the appropriate box to decide which are TRUE and which are FALSE.*

	True	*False*
a) Closed questions are very useful at the state of the interview.		
b) Open questions enable the patient to respond with his or her own words and ideas - so enabling the service provider to better understand the patient.		
c) A good medical interview starts with open questions and moves towards closed questions.		
d) Closed questions enable you to rule out specific symptoms.		

8. *What kind of open question might be worth asking the patient several times, and why?*

____

____

____

Other verbal skills

In addition to positive non-verbal behaviour and appropriate, respectful questioning, there are a number of additional skills which can be extremely useful when interviewing patients with STD. They can help you to deal supportively with the patient's emotions as well as to gather information effectively.

These are the six skills:

- facilitation
- summarising and checking
- reassurance
- direction
- empathy
- partnership.

Facilitation

Nodding the head and raising the eyebrows are two examples of non-verbal facilitation. Here is an example of spoken facilitation in practice:

Patient:	*I'm not sure... it's embarrassing.*
Service provider:	*That's all right, I'm listening.*
Patient:	*Well, it's that...*
Service provider:	Yes?
Patient:	There 's *this sore...*

The service provider can use words, phrases or other sounds to encourage the patient to continue speaking.

Direction

This is a useful approach when a patient is confused and doesn't know where to begin, or when they are talking quickly and mixing up issues of concern.

Patient:	*I don't know, it's been there for three weeks. What am I going to tell my husband? Will anyone get to know? I mean, it is curable isn 't it?*
Service provider:	*Let's find out what the problem is first. We can deal with that, and then we can talk about your husband.*

Direction relieves the frustration of the service provider and allows the patient to share concerns and worries more easily.

Summarising and checking

Summarising and checking allow you to ensure you have understood the patient correctly. The patient is also able to correct any misunderstanding.

Service provider:	(Summarising) *So you're worried what to say to your husband,* and you *feel* very *embarrassed about this condition. You want to know whether we can* cure *it.* (Checking) *Have I got that right?*
Patient:	*That's right. What is wrong with me?*

Use this skill when the patient has mentioned a number of things that you want to confirm .

Empathy

This may be the most important skill of all when dealing with the patient's feelings. Upon noticing that a patient is tense or anxious, for example, you can express your empathy by commenting on what you have noticed:

Service provider: I *can see that this is worrying you a good deal.*
Patient: Yes, *it's been bothering me for over a week now I'm worried sick.*

By showing empathy, you allow the patient to express his or her fears, and establish more open communication between you. Like facilitation, it encourages the patient to continue speaking.

Reassurance

While no-one likes to be patronised with expressions like "Don't worry, it will be all right", reassurance is important to show that you accept the patient's feelings and that the problem need not last forever:

Service provider: I *can understand that you feel worried about symptoms like these. As soon as I confirm what's wrong with you, we can try to begin treatment that will make you better.*
Patient: *That's good. So what else do you need to know?*

Partnership

This skill enables you to offer the patient a commitment - with you personally or the team of people you work with:

Service provider: *You've done the right thing to come here for treatment. Before you leave I'll make quite sure you know everything you need to about preventing further infection. And we'll also find the best way to discuss this with your husband.*
Patient: *Oh thank you. I don't want this to happen again.*

Most good service providers use some of these interviewing skills some of the time. The key to interviewing patients who may have an STD is to use all six skills most of the time. To help you become more familiar with them, try identifying each skill in the interview on the next page.

9. *Please try to identify the different skills that the service provider is using in the case-study below. Underline each example you identify, and say which skill it is in the column on the right.*

Service provider: *Good morning. Please sit down... My name's Lynn Solent. You are?*

Patient: *John Smith.*

Service provider: *How can I help you Mr. Smith?*

Patient: *Well, I cut my arm yesterday while I was pulling out an old tree stump. Look, the cut's quite deep.*

Service provider: *Oh, it's not too bad, but you did the right thing to come and get it cleaned up, Mr. Smith. I can clean and dress it for you easily... Have you come far to have this dressed?*

Patient: *Oh, I live 5 miles away, near {mentions a village}.*

Service provider: *Fine. [Cleans and dresses the wound.}*

Service provider: *Now, is there anything else bothering you Mr. Smith?*

Patient: *Well.... there is something else {he laughs nervously).*

Service provider: *I can see you feel a little embarrassed about this...*

Patient: *Yes I do... you see, it's my {leans forward and whispers} it's my penis.*

Service provider: *Yes?*

Patient: *Well, there's a...there's a sort of.... sore on it.*

Service provider: *And you're worried about this sore.*

Patient: *Yes I am. You see, I didn't cut myself or anything. It doesn't hurt but it doesn't look good. It's worrying me a bit. I mean, one of my girlfriends said it's... well, it's a bad thing and she wouldn't go with me... I think it might have come from a bar girl, or maybe even one of my girlfriends.*

Service provider: *Tell me about this sore.*

Patient: *What's to tell? It doesn't hurt.....(shrugs}.*

Service provider: *How long have you had it?*

Patient: *Oh, a month or so I suppose My uncle says it's nothing to worry about but I think it's from a woman... if I find out which one...*

Service provider: *You're clearly anxious about where you got this sore, Mr. Smith but I think we need to decide what it is first. I think we'll also need to talk about how to prevent it happening again... But first I'll need to examine the sore. . .*

Patient: *{Looks surprised).*
Service provider: *I know this can be embarrassing but I need to do that in order to decide what's wrong. Is that all right with you?*
Patient: *Yes, I suppose so {reluctantly).*
Service provider: *Before I can give you any treatment I must be sure...*
Patient: *It's going to be OK isn't it?*
Service provider: *Oh yes, and I know we can help you to cure it completely. You need to prevent it happening again, but I'll tell you everything you need to know and help you decide what you're going to do about it. Is that OK?*
Patient- *Oh yes.*

Summary

In this section, we have explored good interviewing skills in some detail. We have suggested when and how you might use open and closed questions during the interview, and we have suggested six additional skills and a number of tips to help you meet the interview's objectives: to gather information effectively in the time available and to deal supportively with the patient's feelings.

By now, you should be able to:

- appreciate the importance of demonstrating your respect for each STD patient, by your welcome, the privacy and confidentiality you offer and your respect for their opinions and views;
- keep your questions free of moral judgement;
- use the patient's terms, or words that he or she understands easily;
- request permission to ask personal questions or examine the patient;
- distinguish between open and closed questions;
- identify when to use an open or closed question;
- recognise six additional verbal skills that will help you gather information and support the patient effectively:

  — facilitation
  — direction
  — summarising and checking
  — empathy
  — reassurance
  — partnership.

In the next section, you will learn what information you need to obtain when taking a patient's history. The activity at the end of the section will enable you to put everything you have learned together by practising taking someone's history.

D. STD INFORMATION GATHERING

Having explored the communication skills we need when interviewing a patient with STD, in this short section we will outline the information that we need to gather when taking the patient's history.

You will learn:

- what general information you need to gather, and why it is necessary;
- how to match the information you need to the questioning skills you have learned about.

First, why do we need to take a patient's history? At the start of Section 1, we mentioned three aims:

1. To make a syndromic diagnosis of STD which is accurate and efficient, given the time available.
2. To establish the patient's risk of contracting or transmitting STD.
3. To find out about partners who may have been infected.

Information gathering

To meet these three aims when taking the history of an STD patient, we need to gather information about four areas:

1. General details about the patient.
2. The patient's present illness.
3. His or her medical history.
4. His or her sexual history.

On the next page is a list of the key information you need in each of these areas.

History-taking information

1. General details:
   - Age
   - Number of children
   - Locality or address
   - Employment

2. Present illness:
   - Presenting complaints and duration

Men:

- If an inguinal bubo - Is *it painful? Associated with genital ulcer? Swellings elsewhere in the body?*
- If a urethral discharge - *Pain while passing urine? Frequency?*
- If scrotal swelling - *History of trauma?*

Women:

- If a vaginal discharge - *Pain while passing urine? Frequency?* Risk assessment positive?*
- Lower abdominal pain - *Vaginal bleeding or discharge?* Painful or difficult pregnancy or childbirth? Painful or difficult or irregular menstruation? Missed or overdue period?

Men and women:

- If a genital ulcer - Is *it painful? Recurrent? Appearance?* Spontaneous onset?
- Other symptoms, such as itching or discomfort

3. Medical history

- Any past STD - Type? *Dates? Any treatment and re* sponse? Results of tests?
- Other illness - *Type? Dates? Any treatment and re*sponse? Results of tests?
- Medications
- Drug allergies

4. Sexual history

- Currently active sexually?
- New partner in the last three months?
- Risk assessment*

The reason for asking each of these questions will become cleaner when you have worked through the syndromic flow-charts with Workbook 4.

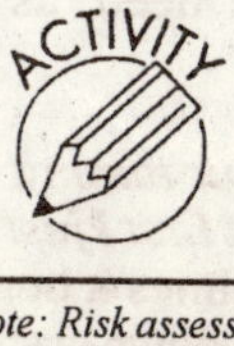

Please read through the information opposite carefully. Note down anything that surprises you or any questions you want to) ask.

---

* *Note: Risk assessment is a specific set of quesfons used for women patients who complain of vaginal discharge. It was devised to help providers decide where the* t *infection is localised.*

Workbook 4 will explain what specific information you need to identify each syndrome, including risk assessment, so many of your questions will be answered then. But please discuss anything with your supervisor or colleagues now if you can.

How do you ask questions to obtain this information?

Next, you need to consider *how you* will ask questions to obtain this information. It would be easy to convert the information on back page into closed questions but, as you know, that means a lot of questions to ask! For example, just to gather information relating to a female patient's abdominal pain, you would have to ask all these closed questions:

- Do you have pain in the lower abdomen?
- Do you have pain when you have sexual intercourse?
- Do you have an unusual vaginal discharge?
- When did you last have your monthly period?
- Was the period unusual in any way?
- Are your periods regular?
- Are they painful?
- Have you missed a period?
- Are you late for a period?

On the other hand, one or two open questions might encourage the patient to provide most of the information you need, as we illustrated in the last section.

Service provider:	*Tell me about this pain in your tummy.*
Patient:	*Well, it started a week ago. At first I just felt tender down here,* but sometimes it begins to hurt a *lot.* It hurts when I sit *down or* stand up - it isn 't like m) *monthly pain at all.*

Service provider: *What else is troubling you?*
Patient: *Well, there is one other thing. There's a* funny *kind of discharge that I don 't usually get. It doesn 't hu rt but it's ... well ... it smells.*

Service provider: *How are your periods?*
Patient: *OK I think. I* mean *I'm regular, and they give me a little pain. But this is different.*

---

10. Now try devising a few *questions that you might ask to* obtain information about a patient's sexual behaviour.

a) First write two or three OPEN questions.

b) Next, write some CLOSED questions you could ask if the patient did not provide you with sufficient information in answer to the open questions. Remember the principles of supportive questioning that we explored in Section-C.!

11. At this point, it's worth looking again at the difficulty of discussing questions like these.

a) Would you feel uncomfortable asking any of the questions you have just written down? If so, why?

b) How would you feel if the patient was older or younger than you? Why?

c) Why do you think the information about sexual history is last on the list on page 20?

Summary

In this third *section,* we have listed the *information you may need to* collect in order to diagnose an STD and also *to* educate the patient and manage their partner or partners. We have also suggested how you could use open and close questions to gather this information.

With your colleagues:

- *if you have not already done so, please discuss your answers to questions 8 and 9.*
- *discuss all the culturally acceptable ways of addressing a man or a woman of different ages.*

- *look again at the list of required information and discuss the language and terminolcgy that patients might use to express such terms.*

- *consider the words people use to describe sexual activity, casual sex and sex workers.*

Skills practice: role-play exercise

The only way to refine your communication skills is to practise them, so this activity is a very important one. If you are studying as part of a course, then your tutor will organise the activity for you. If you are studying on your own or with an informal group, please ask two colleagues to practise with you.

The idea is that one person takes the part of an STD patient, while a second person practises the role of service provider. A third person can observe the interaction and provide feedback the service provider. There should be at least three 'interviews' in all, so that each of you has the opportunity to take on all three roles.

The objectives of the exercise are to:

- *practise communication skills for interviewing patients, so that you can interview real STD patients with more confidence;*
- *practise gathering the relevant information listed on back page*
- *become more aware of your strengths in communication, and have a clear idea of any areas you want to work on further.*

If you are studying with a group and tutor, then your tutor will manage this role-play exercise. Please ask for his or her guidance on what to do.

ACTIVITY

THE THREE ROLES

The patient's role

Your role is to take the part of a patient with STD who has attended the health facility for treatment. Please decide who you are and what your character is: the questions below may help you. Don't let your interviewer see these notes in advance! Make the patient as realistic as you can: try to BE this person, responding honestly to the person interviewing you. Try not to make it easy or difficult for your interviewer.

What is your name? ______________________

Your sex and age? ______________________

Describe your personality:
outgoing or shy, and so on? ______________________

Describe your beliefs, religion,
education, occupation. ______________________

What STD symptoms do you have?
Anything else? ______________________

How many sexual partners do you have? ______________________

If you have just one sexual partner,
do you know whether he/she
has any other sexual partners? ______________________

How do you feel about the
health facility you are visiting? ______________________

How do you feel about your
symptoms, and about
discussing them with someone else? ______________________

After the role play, give your interviewer feedback on how well they have done. Concentrate especially on how you felt as the patient: to what extent did the interviewer make you feel comfortable, or put you at ease? Did they gain all the information about you that you had noted down?

The observer

The observer's role is a very important one because you are going to give the 'interviewer' objective feedback on the skills they have demonstrated during the role-play. As you observe, use the checklist below to make notes on what the interviewer does.

In giving feedback to the interviewer, try to be as objective and helpful as you can. Be clear about what he or she has done well, and explain why. Also, be willing to criticise the interview r, but in a positive way: in terms of what he or she needs to practise or refine.

Observation checklist–

Does the interviewer:

Treat the patient with respect?

Show he/she is listening by appropriate non-verbal behaviour?

Obtain the patient's permission to ask awkward, embarrassing questions?

Deal effectively with the patient's emotions?

Use mainly open questions, limiting the number of closed questions?

Use these six verbal skills effectively?

- *facilitation*
- *direction*
- *summarising and checking*
- *empathy*
- *reassurance*
- *partnership.*

Ask questions relating to the four areas of information required?

The service provider

During the role-play, be yourself. Try to use all the verbal and nonverbal skills explored in the workbook, keeping in touch with what the patient is feeling and responding to these emotions. Try also to obtain as much appropriate information about the patient as you can in about five minutes.

While the 'patient' is defining who he/she is, you might to look over the observer's checklist to see the sort of skills you are expected to practise.

After the interview, you will receive feedback from the patient and then from the observer. The observer will concentrate on your skills as listed on his or her checklist, while the patient will describe how he/she felt during the interview. He/she will also tell you if you missed anything important about him or her!

E. EXAMINATION

The purpose of a physical examination is to confirm any STD symptoms the patient has described by checking for signs of STD.

This section explains what to do when examining male and female patients. Examining the most private parts of a person's body requires tact, sensitivity and respect on the part of the service provider. Patients may be embarrassed or uncomfortable: this section also suggests ways to help the patient understand the importance of an examination and overcome his or her embarrassment.

This final section will help you to:

- behave professionally with the patient before and during the examination;
- reassure the patient who is reluctant to be examined and gain their confidence and co-operation;
- conduct an efficient examination of both male and female patients.

To get started, please spend a few minutes on these questions.

QUESTION

12. What resources do you need to conduct an examination?

13. What fears do people have about being examined?

14. What must you do in order to reassure all patients before an examination?

These questions raised a number of important points. People may be shy and even reluctant to have their genitals examined, so we must be very professional in our behaviour:

- ensure privacy;
- explain what you are going to do, and why an examination is important;
- even though you may have little time to examine the patient, never be rough with him or her;
- approach the examination in a confident and professional way;
- use all the communication skills you have refined with Sections C and D.

For most syndromes, the examination is important in order to arrive at a diagnosis. However, we must never force someone to be examined. So what can you say to a patient who is unwilling to be examined?

---

15. Consider these situations: what might you do or say to persuade the patient to be examined?

a) A patient of the same sex as the service provider refuses to be examined, saying that he or she has clearly explained what is wrong already.

b) A young woman is afraid to say anything, but communicates non-verbally that she is unhappy about being examined.

c) A male patient is reluctant to be examined by a female service provider.

Summary so far

So far, we have explored issues in preparing patients for the examination:

- privacy is essential;
- treat the patient with respect and behave in a culm, friendly and professional manner, as during the rest of the interview;
- avoid showing your own embarrassment or shyness;
- If the service provider is male, offer female patients the opportunity to have, someone else present if they prefer;
- explain to reluctant patients why you need to examine them.

Next, we will provide you with clear steps on how to examine male and female patients. Your development activity at the end of the workbook will then enable you to put what you have learned into practice - essential to perform an effective examination in the short time you have available.

1. *Syndromic diagnosis of STD in female patients only requires inspection of the external genitals, so gloves are not essential. For signs such as inguinal buboes, gloves are optional.*
2. *As elsewhere in the STD case management programme, this section focuses on examination for seven STD syndromes only. It does not take account of STD such as scabies or lice, treatment of which should be a normal part of your responsibilities. .*

Examining male patients for STD syndromes

1. Ask the patient to stand up and lower his pants so that he is stripped from the chest down to the knees. It may be possible to examine him while he is standing up, though you will sometimes find it easier if the patient lies down.
2. Palpate the inguinal region in order to detect the presence or absence of enlarged lymph nodes and buboes.
3. Palpate the scrotum, feeling for individual parts of the anatomy:
   - testes;
   - spermatic cord.
   - epididymis;
4. Examine the penis, noting any rashes or sores. Then ask the patient to retract the foreskin if present, and look at the:
   - glans penis;
   - urethral meutus.

If you cannot see an obvious urethral discharge, ask the patient to milk the urethra in order to express any discharge.

5. Record the presence or absence of:
   - buboes;
   - urethral discharge, noting the colour and amount.
   - ulcers;

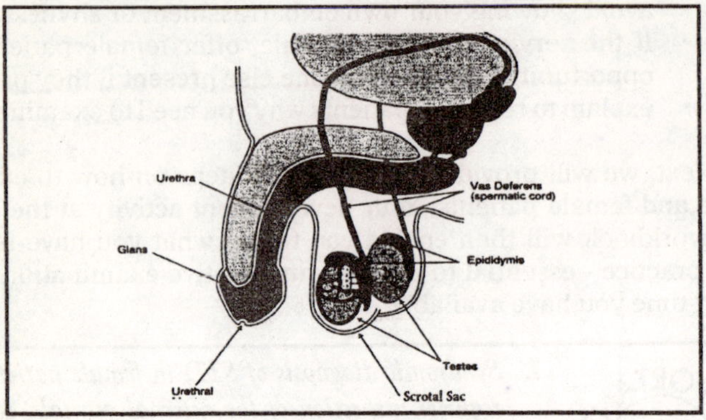

Examining female patients for STD syndromes

1. Ask the patient to remove her clothing from the chest down, and then to lie on the couch. In order to save her embarrassment, use a sheet to cover the parts of the body that you are not examining.
2. Ask the patient to bend her knees and separate her legs, then examin the vulva, anus and perineum.
3. Palpate the inguinal region in order to detect the presence or absence of enlarged lymph nodes and buboes.
4. Palpate the abdomen for pelvic masses and tenderness, taking great care not to hurt the patient.
5. Record the presence or absence of:
   - buboes;
   - ulcers;
   - vaginal discharge, noting the type, colour and amount.

Gloves are required if you wish to conduct a vaginal or bimanual examination .

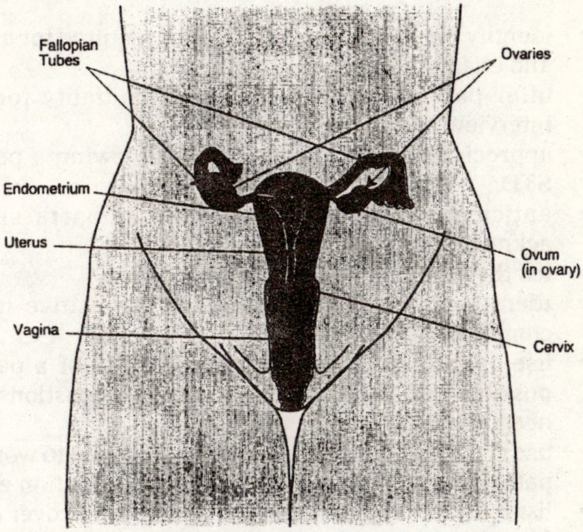
Fallopian Tubes
Ovaries
Endometrium
Uterus
Ovum (in ovary)
Vagina
Cervix

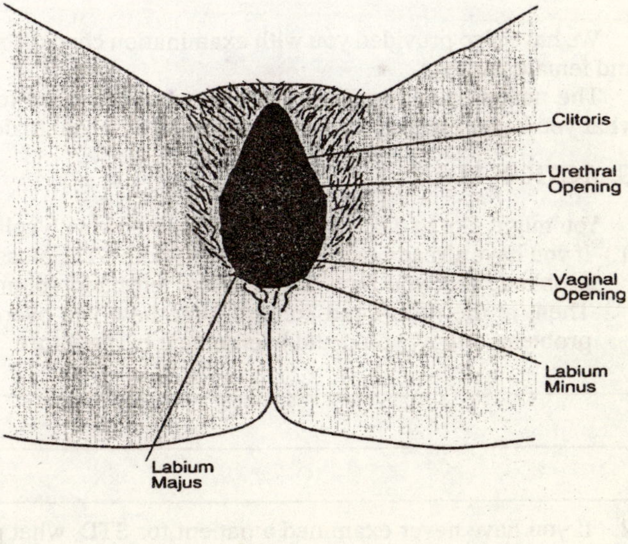
Clitoris
Urethral Opening
Vaginal Opening
Labium Minus
Labium Majus

F. REVIEW

Now that you have completed Workbook 3, you should be able to:

- identify the resources and facilities required for questioning and examine patients;
- offer patients privacy and confidentiality for both the interview and the examination;
- appreciate the uniqueness of interviewing a patient with STD;
- anticipate patients' anxiety and embarrassment, and acknowledge your own feelings;
- list three aims of the interview;
- identify four essential features of positive non-verbal communication;
- use open questions to take the history of a patient with possible STD, following up with closed questions when you need to obtain specific details
- use six further verbal skills that enable you to work with the patient's feeling in order to gather information effectively;
- list four areas of information you need to cover during the interview;
- conduct an efficient examination of both male and female patients;
- reassure the patient who is reluctant to be examined and gain their compliance.

We have also provided you with examination checklists for male and female patients .

The next step is very important because you need to practise what you have learned. The action plan will help you to do this.

G. ACTION PLAN

You might like to discuss the questions below with colleagues.

1. If you have already examined patients with STD, please list any problems that you have faced in the left-hand column below. Then, in the right-hand column, note how you overcame the problem, or how you could overcome it in the future.

---

2. If you have never examined a patient for STD, what problems do you foresee, and how might you overcome it?

____

____

____

3. Discuss the facilities at your health centre: to what extent is it possible to offer STD patients privacy and confidentiality? If necessary, what can you do to improve this situation?

4. You can only learn or refine these skills by practising them. So, if you have practised role-plays with colleagues, over the next few weeks practise history-taking and examination on real patients. Aim to conduct about six of each, and make notes on how you are doing, using the space on the next page. Aim to feel confident in your skills by the time you have completed the action plan.

____

Action plan record: history-taking and examination

Name of clinic:

History taken on (date):	Problems/successes (consider diagnostic and personal skills)
1. ______________	______________
	______________
2. ______________	______________
	______________
3. ______________	______________
	______________
4. ______________	______________
	______________
5. ______________	______________
	______________
6. ______________	______________
	______________

Examination carried out on (date):

1. ______________	______________
	______________

2. ____________________ ____________________

____

3. ____________________ ____________________

____

4. ____________________ ____________________

____

5. ____________________ ____________________

____

6. ____________________ ____________________

____

H. ANSWERS

1. There are no right or wrong answers to this question. Some people will feel nervous, embarrassed, anxious, ashamed or even horrified - as you might do yourself if you were a patient. The strength of such feelings might depend on the patient's awareness of STD or their beliefs about the cause of their symptoms, on their gender, age or social status, or even on whether or not they know the service provider. In fact, the answers to this question could be, as many and varied as the people who attend the health centre.
   An important outcome of these anxious feelings is that people rarely present with the symptoms causing most concern. A patient with a genital ulcer or discharge will often complain of a headache or sore throat at first. Discovering the real symptoms depends on the skills, attitude and encouragement of the service provider!
2. Our reason for asking the second question was to look at the interview from a different perspective: the feelings of the service *provider*. It is not only patients who may be embarrassed or anxious, because the questions we have to ask are very personal ones. Sexuality is private and personal to the individual. It is important that you acknowledge your own feelings about asking such personal questions so that you can work positively and sympathetically with all your patients.
3. Amina's behaviour is likely to make anyone feel small and unimportant like a child who's found doing something wrong. But how each individual would feel depends on their character. An assertive person might feel angry with Amina, whereas a more shy person might be scared. Given that this patient already seems embarrassed by her symptoms, there's little likelihood of a successful interview!

4. So what did Amina do? It is not difficult to criticise her. You may have found even more points than in this list:
   - Amina doesn't greet the patient at all, or introduce herself;
   - she barely looks at the patient for the first few minutes;
   - she begins talking while someone else is still in the room;
   - she speaks and behaves in an impatient, unfriendly manner;
   - she shows no sympathy for the patient's embarrassment-indeed, she becomes more irritated: "Goodness me! I haven't got all day!"

Unfortunately, most of us can remember the odd occasion when we've been treated like that by someone ...

5. Don't worry if you found this activity difficult, specially if you have not had any previous training in interviewing. We wanted to raise these points:

   a) *At the start of the interview:*
   "Name?"
   This is not a friendly way to begin questioning anyone. We should always be polite: "What is your name?" or "Tell me your name please". And why not introduce *yourself* to the client?

   b) *"Tell me your medical history.*
   " This question is too vague. The patient does not know where to begin what a medical history is or what aspects of their history you wont to know about. We need to make our questions more precise.

   c) *"How many sexual partners have you had, when, and who are they?*
   A difficult question to ask in any event, but in this case it is very difficult to answer because there are three questions! Ask only one question at a time. Another tip - when you begin asking deeply personal questions, begin by asking the patient's *permission.* Acknowledge that the question will be hard to answer: the patient will feel you understand his or her feelings better.

   d) *"Have* you *had sex with people other than your husband?"*
   This question suggests a moral judgement on the part of the service provider. We need to make our questions free of such judgements whenever possible.

   e) *"The symptoms only recur during your periods, don't they?"*

This question puts words in the patient's mouth! It is known as a 'leading' question. Avoid it. "When do you get this problem?" or "What makes the problem worse?" would be better.

f) *"Are your menses normal?"*
The tip here is to avoid using medical expressions that the patient might not know. Better to ask the patient what is troubling them or how you can help them.

6. if you remember that closed questions can be answered in one short phrase or with 'yes' and 'no', then this question should be easy. There are only three open quest.ons:

Do you have a *discharge?*- Closed
Are you married?- Closed
What is troubling you?- Open
Is it painful? - Closed
Did you use *a condom last* time you *had* sex? - Closed
Is the *discharge milky or clear?*- Closed
What *does* the *pain feel like?*- Open
Tell me about your periods. - Open

7. a) *Closed questions are very useful* at the start *of the interview.*
FALSE: although closed questions require a specific answer, it is not true that they are useful at the start of the interview: on the contrary avoid them!

b) *Open questions enable* the *patient* to *respond* with their *own* words *and ideas, and give* the *service provider a good understanding of their perceptions.*
TRUE: this is one of the benefits of using open questions at the start of the interview. They enable you to gather information quickly and efficiently, to collect important information you might otherwise have missed, and to learn about the patient's perceptions, concerns and language - all of which will be important later if you need to educate the patient about STD.

c) *A good medical interview starts with open questions and moves towards closed questions.*
TRUE: remember the open-close triangle. We discussed the benefits of open questions early in the interview. The value of closed questions lies in checking or obtaining specific details later in the interview.

d) Closed *questions enable you to rule out specific symptoms.*
TRUE: by asking closed questions you can rule out specific symptoms but remember to start with open questions at the beginning of the interview.

8. Don't worry if you forgot this one: we were thinking of asking the patient " anything more troubling you?", or a question to that effect. The reason why such questions are so important is that they allow the patient who feels nervous or anxious to work towards their main and most private concerns their own way. Remember that many patients with STD symptoms will feels embarrassed by them that they will feel reluctant to admit to such symptoms until you have demonstrated your willingness to listen and treat them with respect.

9. We have marked the main skills that Lynn is using on the next page. Please discuss your findings with a colleague or tutor if you are not sure about anything in this exercise.
   You might also like to discuss anything else that Lynn could have said or done for this patient ...

Service provider:	*Good morning. Please sit down ... My name's Lyn Solent. You are?*	*An open question facilitation*
Patient:	*John Smith.*	
Service provider:	*How can I help you Mr. Smith?*	*Open question*
Patient:	*Well, I cut my arm yesterday while I was pulling out an old tree stump. Look, the cut's quite deep.*	
Service provider:	*Oh, it's not too bad. But you did the right thing to come and get it cleaned up, Mr. Smith. I can clean and dress it for you easily... Have you come tar to have this dressed?*	*Reassurance*
Patient:	*Oh, I live 5 miles away, near {mentions a village.*	
Service provider:	*Fine. {Cleans and dresses the wound.}*	
Service provider:	*Now, is there anything else bothering. you Mr. Smith ?*	*Open, facilitation*
Patient:	*Well... there is something else the laughs nervously.*	
Service provider:	*I can see you feel a little*	

	embarrassed about this...	*Empathy*
Patient:	*Yes I do... you see, it's my {leans forward and whispers)... it's my penis.*	
Service provider:	*Yes?*	*Facilitation*
Patient:	*Well, there's a... there's a sort of... sore on it.*	
Service provider:	*And you 're worried about this sore.*	*Empathy checking*
Patient:	*Yes I am. You see, I didn't cut myself or anything. It doesn't hurt but it doesn't look good. It's worrying me a bit. I mean, one of my girl friends said it is well, it's a bad thing and she wouldn't go with me... I think it might have come from a bar girl, or maybe even one of my girlfriends.*	
Service provider:	*Tell me about this sore.*	*Open direction*
Patient:	*What's to tell? It doesn't hurt... {shrugs).*	
Service provider:	*How long. have you had it?*	*Closed, used to facilitation*
Patient:	*Oh, a month or so I suppose. My uncle says it's nothing to worry about but I think it's from a woman... if I find out which one...*	
Service provider:	*You're clearly anxious about where you got this sore Mr. Smith. But I think we need to decide what it is first. I think we '11 also need to talk about how to prevent it happening again... But first I'll need to examine the sore...*	*Direction*
Patient.	*(Looks surprised).*	
Service provider:	*I know this can be, embarrassing. but I need to do* at in order to decide what's wrong Is tha' all *right with you?*	*Reassurance, checking*
Patient:	*Yes, I suppose so {reluctantly).*	
Service provider:	*A sore might mean a very dangerous disease, so I must be sure...*	

Patient:	*It's going to be OK isn 't it?*	*Reassurance,*
Service provider:	*Oh yes, and I know we can help you to cure it completely. You need to prevent it appearing again. But I'll tell you everything you need to know and help you decide what you regoing to do about it. Is that OK?*	*partnership* *Checking*
Patient:	*Oh yes.*	

10. There can't be any right or wrong answers to this question - just slightly better or worse ones, so please discuss your own questions with colleagues. The case study listed below is only intended as a rough guide to how an interview on sexual history might go. Notice how the service provider starts this part of the interview, and how closed questions are used only to get specific information. The patient is also reassured and praised for her openness.

Service provider: *I need to ask you a few very personal questions now about your sexuality. I know this is difficult to talk about, but I assure you no-one else will know.*
Patient: *Why* does that *matter* to you?
Service provider: *That's a good question. It's party to help me make sure I'm giving you the right treatment, and party to help us know how many people might have the same infection. Is that OK?*
Patient: *... Yes ... all right.*
Service provider: *Have you been sexually active over the last 3 months or* so?
Patient: *Well, yes, I suppose* so.
Service provider: *Tell me about that.*
Patient: *What* do you *want to know?*
Service provider: *Oh, how often, who with, that sort of thing.*
Patient: *Well... I've* got two *boyfriends... Well, there's another friend who I sleep with sometimes but he's usually away...*
Service provider: *When did you last sleep with the friend who's away a lot?*
Patient: *I can't remember... sometimes last month I suppose.*
Service provider: *And what about your other boyfriends?*
Patient: *Well, Ro is my proper boyfriend. We spent the night together two nights ago... well, we often* do...

Service provider:	*What about your other boyfriend?*
Patient:	*Well... Ro doesn't know about the others.*
Service provider:	*That's all right. I promise he needn't know you're being very brave about all this.*
Patient:	*Well. . . I see him every Tuesday. Usually. . . but I didn't see him last Tuesday because I was with my parents then.*
Service provider:	*What do you think of condoms?*
Patient:	*I don't like them wouldn't use one.*
Service provider:	*Do you know if any of your boyfriends has a discharge at the moment?*
Patient:	*No. . . I mean I'm not sure, I don 't know.*
Service provider:	*That's OK. Any other boyfriends in the last 3 months?*
Patient:	*Oh no.*
Service provider:	*That's fine. You've done very well, so now I can tell you what this discharge is....*

11.a] Most people find it uncomfortable asking such personal questions at first. It is quite normal to feel that way. With experience many service providers lose their embarrassment-but few patients do!

b) The answer to this question depends on cultural and social values as well as individual ones. Please compare your answer with those of colleagues if you can.

c) We've commented before that sexuality is difficult to discuss. By asking less difficult questions first, and using effective communication skills, you make time to win the patient's trust *before* asking questions about their sexual history.

12. To conduct an examination, you need:
    - a well-lit, private room;
    - an examination table for the patient to lie on for the examination, and a chair;
    - time! This may also limit the extent of the physical examination. Managing an STD patient can take anything from 5 to 15 minutes. In one African country, for example, service providers spend only 5 or 6 minutes with each patient. In another country, STD visits in 20 health centres averaged 15 minutes for women and 10 minutes for men - not including waiting time.
13. Most patients will feel very shy about showing their genitals to another person, especially a member of the opposite sex. Some people may also feel ashamed of their symptoms, even though anxiety about the symptoms has brought them to the clinic.
14. The one most important factor in reassuring patients before

examination is that you will ensure them privacy and confidentiality.

15. Remember that you cannot force any person to be examined.
    a) In the first situation, both service provider and patient are the same sex.
        - explain why you want to do the examination, namely that you need to check his/her condition to make sure you give the right treatment;
        - emphasize that the examination will be brief and *not* painful;
    b) Whenever a female patient is being examined by a male service provider, it is a good idea that someone else - a friend or female service provider - is present. This will almost certainly make the situation more comfortable for the woman.
    c) In this circumstance, try persuading the patient with the suggestions listed in 1 5a above. You can also offer to have a male member of staff present in the room while you examine. If this does not work (and perhaps there are strong cultural reasons why a male patient should refuse to be examined by a female service provider), your only alternative is that a male service provider should make the examination.

GLOSSARY

Bubo	Painful inguinal swelling
Closed questions	Questions that only encourage one or two word answers, for example 'Are you married?' (compare with *open questions*)
Direction	One of the six verbal skills - asking patient to focus on one point at a time
Empathy	One of the six verbal skills - commenting on patient's behaviour, so encouraging him/her to express concerns
Epididymis	A duct behind the *testis*, along which sperm passes to the vas deferens
Facilitation	One of the six verbal skills - using words, phrases or sounds to encourage the patient to continue talking
Glans penis	The rounded part forming the end of the penis
Inguina/ region	Groin
Lymph nodes	Small mass of tissue that is part of the Lymphatic system

Menses	Menstruation or the blood and other materials discharged from the uterus at menstruation
Open questions	Questions that invite detailed answers, usually beginning How? What? Where? or Why? (see also *closed questions*)
Palpote	To examine by touch
Partnership	One of the six verbal skills - offering the Patient a commitment, with you or the health team
Pelvic masses	Tumorous growths in the pelvic region
Perineum	The area between the anus and scrotum or *vulva*
Reassurance	One of the six verbal skills - persuading the patient that you accept his or her feelings and that the problem will pass in time
Summarising and checking	Two of the six verbal skills - summarising what patient has said to check that you have understood correctly
Testes	The medical name for testicles
Ulcer	Open sore
Urethral meatus	Opening/possage of the urethra
Vas deferens	Duct that carries sperm from the testicle to the urethra (also called spermatic cord)
Vulva	External female genitals

5

DIAGNOSIS AND TREATMENT

A. INTRODUCTION

This workbook provides you with a practical, step-by-step guide to each of the seven syndromic flow-charts.

For each flow-chart, it explains all the important decision boxes and action boxes and lists all the required drugs and doses recommended by WHO. Whenever possible, it also suggests alternative drug therapies for situations in which those specified are unavailable or ineffective.

At the end of the workbook you will find lots of questions to help you check your understanding of the flow-charts, as well as an action plan that will help you develop your skills.

Your learning objectives

This workbook provides you with all the information you need in order to:

- use the seven flow-charts to diagnose STD accurately;
- give the correct drug therapies and dosages for each diagnosis;
- advise and educate patients on a number of important issues.

For esse of use, there is a copy of the appropriate flow-chart at the top of the first page on each syndrome.

You will find this workbook easier if you have first studied Workbook 2, using flow-charts for Syndromic Management, and Workbook 3, History-Taking and Examination. These two workbooks provide a broad overview of the techniques and skills you need.

Workbooks 5 and 6 deal with patient education and counselling and partner management in detail.

General guidelines on use of the flow-charts.

For each of the syndromic management flow-charts, the following detailed information is provided:

- basic details that are necessary for diagnosis and treatment;
- guidelines on history-taking or examination which are essential to the diagnosis of a particular syndrome;
- the recommended drugs for each diagnosis, including alternatives that are;
  necessary for pregnant or lactating women;
- education or counselling needed for this diagnosis.

The entry-point for each flow-chart

As you already know if you have studied Workbook 2, the entry point to each of the flow-charts is a problem box like this. It contains an STD-related symptom.

Patient complains of vaginal discharge

Workbook 3 explored the skills you need for history-taking and examination. You should be able to turn to the appropriate flow-chart as soon as you have a clear understanding of a patient's symptoms.

The action boxes for each flow-chart

The action boxes ask you to do something. The ones at the end of a flow-chart list basic issues on which you need to educate or advise the patient. They include actions such as these:

* treat for (the cause or causes);
• educate;
• counsel if needed;
* promote/provide condoms;
• partner management.

Drug treatment

The action box contains instructions to treat with drugs for a particular syndrome. All the drugs we suggest in this workbook are recommended by WHO. However, national recommendations may vary from country to country, so use those drugs recommended by your national guidelines.

Educate

- Advise your patient on the importance of complying with treatment, especially in completing a course of tablets. Also explain the mode of transmission of STD and the possible complications of infection. Advise the patient not to engage in sexual activity until completely cured.

- Educate the patient on safer sexual behaviour: abstaining from sexual activity, maintaining a mutually faithful sexual relationship, engaging only in safe sex acts, such as non-penetrative sex or having sex only with condoms. This is a very important issue: take a little time to educate your patient.
- Explain why it is important that the patient's sexual partners should also be treated.

Counsel if needed

Use the communication skills you refined with Workbook 3 to help the patient cope with any anxieties. For example, some people may not feel in a position to refuse a sexual relationship, and they may need to talk about this. (Workbook 5 will help you learn much more about how to educate and support patients with STD.)

Promote/provide condoms

Educate the patient on proper condom use. Demonstrate condom use on a model and either give the patient a supply of condoms or discuss where to get them. Advice on condom use should include safe and hygienic disposal of condoms.

Partner management

This involves more than just asking patients to identify sexual partners. The patient may need your help to decide what to say to partners. You will need to develop special skills in managing people who come to the clinic because their partner has been treated for an STD.

> *Syndromic diagnosis of STD in women does not require internal examination, so gloves are not necessary.*
> *Remember: always treat your patient with courtesy and respect. YOU must win their trust and confidence if you are to provide comprehensive and effective STD case management.*

B. URETHRAL DISCHARGE

A man presents himself to your clinic complaining that he has noticed a discharge from the penis. Use the flow-chart for urethral discharge.

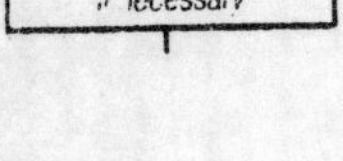

This action box requires you to examine the patient in order to confirm that the patient has a urethral discharge and to see if any other STD is present.

Look at the external genitalia, not forgetting the inner surface of the foreskin and the parts normally covered by the foreskin. If you cannot see any discharge, ask *the patient* to squeeze the penis and milk the urethra. After examining the patient, go to the next box.

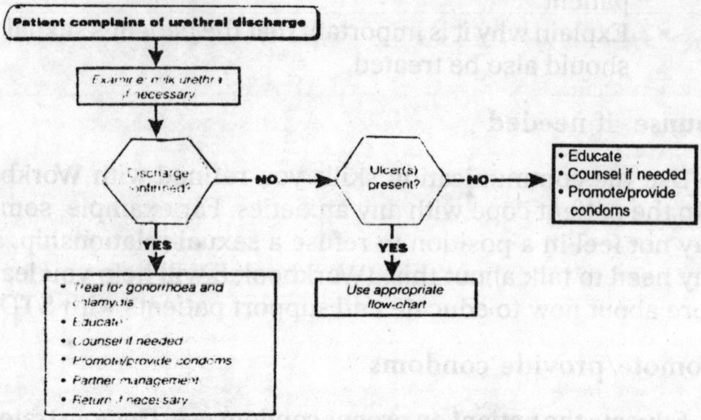

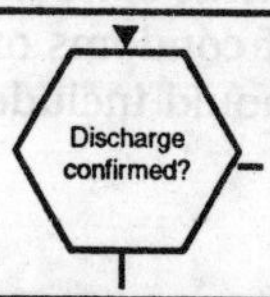

This decision box asks you whether or not there is a urethral discharge. If there is, go to the action box immediately below. If you cannot find a urethral discharge, proceed to the decision box on the right.

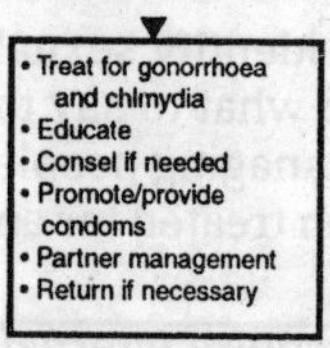

This action box tells you exactly what to do for your patient. Follow all the instructions in the box to deliver comprehensive care. The box tells you what treatment to give and reminds you to educate him, promote condom use and supply them if this is your policy. Also ask the patient to return if he is not better after completing the treatment.

- Treat your patient for gonorrhoea and chlamydial infection.

  — For the treatment of *gonococcal urethritis*, give CIPROFLOXACIN 500 mg in a single oral dose, OR CEFTRIAXONE 250 mg single i.m. dose, OR CEFIXIME 400 mg single oral dose, OR SPECTINOMYCIN 2 g single i.m. dose.

  In regions where kanamycin and cotrimoxazole show continuing efficacy in the treatment of gonorrhoea, these drugs may also be used:

Kanamycin 2 single i.m. dose, OR, when single dose therapy is not available:
Trimethoprim 80 mg/Sulphomethoxazole 400 mg (Cotrimoxazole) 10 tablets orally, once daily for three days.

PLUS

For the treatment of *chlamydial urethritis*, give DOXYCYCLINE 100 mg orally twice daily for seven days OR TETRACYCLINE 500 mg orally four times daily for seven days.

Alternatively, the following drugs may be used: Erythromycin 500 mg orally four times doily for seven days OR Sulfisoxazole 500 mg orally four times daily for 10 days (equivalent doses of other sulphonumides may also be usedl.

- Ask the patient to return in a week's time if his symptoms persist..

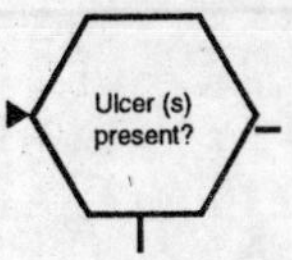

This box asks you to decide whether the patient also has a genital ulcer. If the patient has no evidence of any other STD, go to the box -on the right. If there is evidence of another STD then go to the action box immediately below.

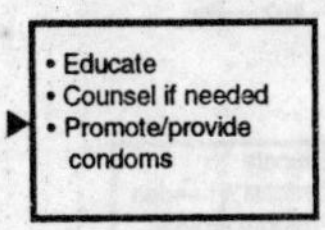

You have not been able to confirm the presence of urethral discharge nor of any other STD. The patient may simply be worried that he may have an STD as a result of taking part in risky sexual behaviour, so this box requires you to reassure your patient, educate him and promote the use of condoms (supplying them if this is your policy).

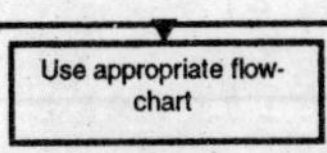

If the Patient has ulcers, simply turn to the flow-chart for genital ulcers

---

Before reading further, check with your supervisor which drugs your facility recommends for treating urethral discharge Make a note of the treatment here:

Now work through the case history below to practise using the flow-chart, then note down what treatment action you will take.

For the lost two days a middle-aged *businessman has hod pain when he posses urine. There is a slight watery discharge* from *the tip* of *his penis. His wife is in the village and he has not seen* her for three months.

Please check your answer with another colleague or your supervisor to make sure that you followed the right pathway through the flow-chart.

C. GENITAL ULCERS

A patient at your clinic complains that he or she has noticed a sore on the genitals use the flow-chart for genital ulcer disease.

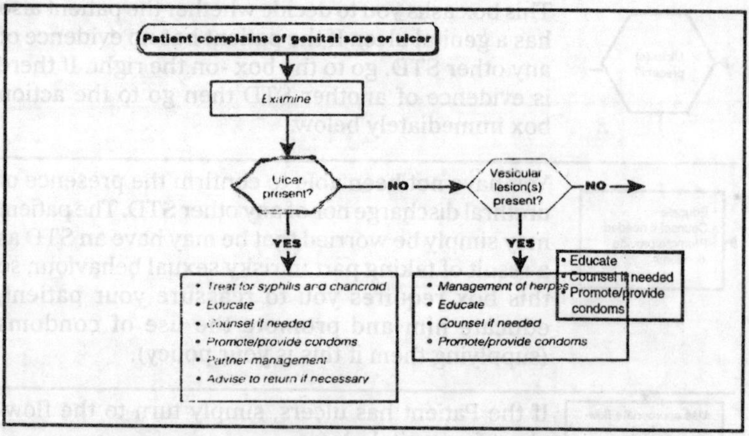

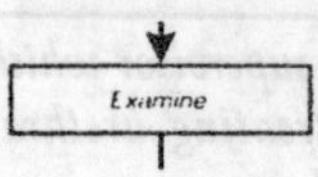

This box asks you to examine the patient for genital ulcer and any other STD that may be present. An ulcer is a break in the continuity of the skin or mucous membrane surface.

- In *men* look at external genitalia, not forgetting the inner surface of the foreskin and the parts normally covered by the foreskin
- In *women* examine the skin of the external genitalia; ask the patient to separate the labia so that you can look at the mucous surfaces for ulcers.

After you have examined the patient, go to the next box.

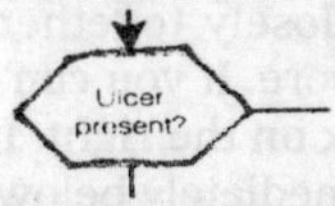

If there is a genital ulcer, go to the action box below. If you cannot find a genital ulcers go the decision box on the right.

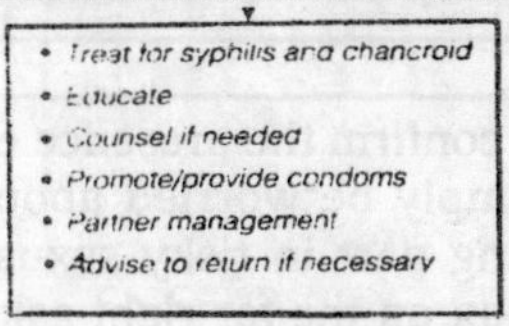

This action box tells you to treat your patient for both syphilis and chancroid. It also tells you to educate him or her, promote the use of condoms and ask the patient to return in seven days if their symptoms have not improved.

- *For the treatment of syphilis,* give the patient BENZATHINE PENICILLIN G 2.4 million units intramuscularly at a single session (because of the volume of this dose, give it as two injections at separate sites).

  For non-pregnant patients who are allergic to penicillin, use: Tetracycline 500 mg orally four times daily for 15 days, OR Doxycycline 100 mg orally twice daily for 15 days, OR Erythromycin 500 mg orally four times daily for 10 days, OR Sulfisoxazole 500 mg orally four times daily for 10 days equivalent doses of other sulphonsmides may also be used).

  NOTE: Ciprofloxacin, doxycycline and tetracycline should not be used during pregnancy or lactation.

PLUS

- For the treatment of *chancroid,* give ERYTHROMYCIN 500 mg orally three times doily for seven days.

  Alternatively, the following may be used:
  Ciprofloxacin 500 mg single oral dose, OR
  Cehrioxone 250 mg single i.m. dose, OR
  Spectinomycin 2 9 single i.m. dose or, in places where continuing efficacy has been demonstrated Trimethoprim 80 mg/Sulphamethoxazole 400 mg (Cotrimoxazole) two tablets orally, twice daily for seven days.

- Advise the patient to take all the tablets and inform him or her about the mode of transmission of STD and possible complications of infection.

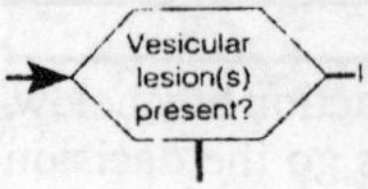

If no ulcer is present, this second decision box asks if vesicular lesions are present. They look like a number of tiny blisters packed closely together, before they burst to form a small sore. If you can't see any such lesions, go to the box on the right. If they are present, go to the box immediately below.

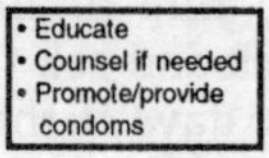

You have not been able to confirm the presence of STD. The patient may simply be worried about having an STD after taking part in risky sexual behoviour, so the action box on the far right asks you to reassure your patient, educate him or her and promote the use of condoms supplying them if this is your policy).

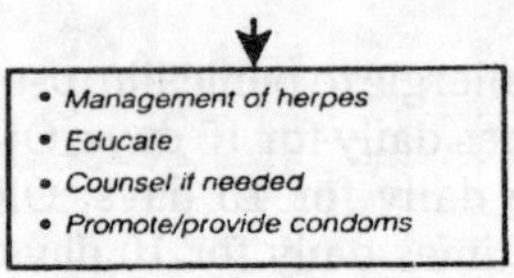

This right-hand action box asks you to educate the patient on the management of herpes. Reassure him or her that, although the lesions cannot be cured, they will go away (but might recur) of their own accord. Explain the importance of keeping the area clean and dry, and advise the patient not to have sex until the area has healed.

ACTIVITY

Before reading further, check with your supervisor which drugs your facility recommends for treating genital ulcers. Make a note of the treatment here:

Now work through the case history below to practise using the flow-chart, then note down what treatment action you will take.

A young woman complains of a painful vulva. Her husband is her only partner. She appears ill and feverish. On examination, she has many small sores filled with a clear liquid on both labia majora and minora, and no visible ulcer.

Please check your answer with another colleague or your supervisor to *make sure that you followed the right pathway through the flow-chart.*

D. VAGINAL DISCHARGE

It is normal for women to have some vaginal discharge. This is known as a Physiologic discharge. It may be more pronounced during certain phases of the menstrual cycle, during and after sexual activity and during pregnancy and aftion. Usually women complain of vaginal discharge only when they perceive It as being unusual for them or if it causes itching or discomfort. In general they will not seek medication for a physiological discharge.

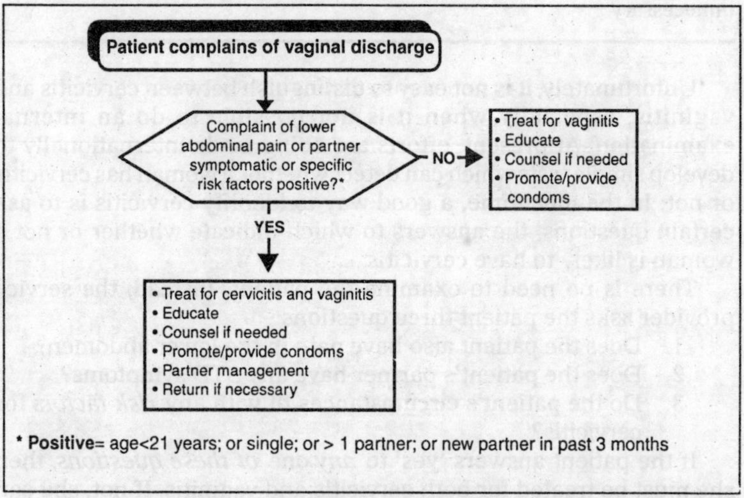

Women develop the symptom of vaginal discharge if they have either vaginitis (infection of the vagina) or cervicitis (infection of the cervix), or both. It is useful. to distinguish between these conditions because one of them, cervicitis, leads to serious complications, therefore, a patient's sexual partner(s) must also be treated.

We can summaries the differences between vaginitis and cervicitis with this table.

Vaginitis	*Cervicitis*
Caused by trichomoniasis, candidiasis and bacterial vaginosis	Caused by gonorrhoea and chlamydia
Most common cause of voginal discharge	Less common cause of vaginal discharge
Easy to diagnose	Difficult to diagnose
No complications	Major complications
Treatment of partner unnecessary	Need to treat partner

Unfortunately, it is not easy to distinguish between cervicitis and vaginitis, especially when it is not possible to do an internal examination. At present, efforts are being made internationally to develop simple tests which can detect whether a woman has cervicitis or not; In the meantime, a good way to identify cervicitis is to ask certain questions, the answers to which indicate whether or not a woman is likely to have cervicitis.

There is no need to examine the patient. Instead, the service provider asks the patient three questions:

1. Does the patient also have pain in the lower abdomen?
2. Does the patient's partner have any STD symptoms?
3. Do the patient's circumstances fit with any *risk factors* for cervicitis?

If the patient answers 'yes' to *any* one *of these questions,* then she must be treated for both cervicitis and vaginitis. If not, she can be treated for vaginitis alone.

The first two questions are straightforward, but what about the third one? What are these risk factors?

The risk factors

Studies in a number of African countries have identified four risk factors which are effective in predicting cervicitis. They are:

- patient is aged less than 21 years;
- patient is single;
- patient has had sex with more than one person in the preceding three months;
- patient has had sex with a new partner in the preceding three months.

To diagnose cervicitis as well as vaginitis, *any one or more of* these risk factors or the first two questions above must be positive.

Remember: The risk factors above were developed for, and apply to, countries in Africa. They will need to be adapted for other countries. If necessary, your trainer or supervisor will provide you with adapted risk factors.

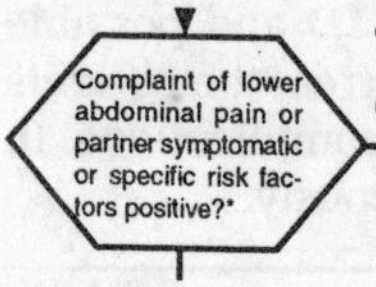

This decision box asks you to question the patient on three issues:

1. Is the patient's sexual partner symptomatic?
2. Does the patient also complain of lower abdominal pain?
3. Does one of these risk factors apply to this patient:
   - less than 21 years of age?
   - single?
   - more than one sexual partner in the last three months?
   - a new sexual partner in the last three months?

If the patient answers YES to any one of these questions, she and her partner must be treated for both cervicitis and vaginitis. Move to the action box below.

If the patient responds negatively to all questions, she can be treated for vaginitis only. Move to the action box at next page.

With your tutor or supervisor, work out a way to ask these questions so that patients can easily understand them. For example, a way to ask about a new sexual partner in the last three months could be: "Have you had a new sexual partner since Christmas (or some other significant event three months ago)?"

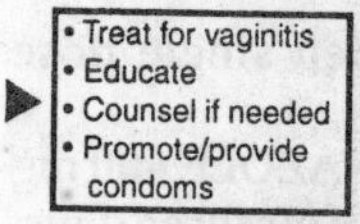

Use this action box if the patient answers NO to all the questions in the vaginal discharge decision box.

Treatment for vaginitis includes treatment for trichomoniasis, candidiasis and bacterial vaginosis:

- For effective treatment for both trichomoniasis and bacterial vaginosis, give METRONIDAZOLE 2 g as a single oral dose to be taken at the clinic under supervision. METRONIDAZOLE 400-500 mg given orally twice daily for seven days is also effective.

  Note: Do not prescribe Metronidazole in the first trimester of pregnancy, and warn the patient against drinking alcohol while taking Metronidazole.

- Effective treatment for VAGINAL CANDIDIASIS is NYSTATIN 100, 000 units (one pessary), inserted intravaginally once a day for 14 days, OR

MICONAZOLE OR CLOTRIMAZOLE 200 mg, inserted into the vagina once a day for three days, OR
CLOTRIMAZOLE 500 mg, inserted into the vagina once only.

- Advise the patient to take the complete course of tablets and inform her of the mode of transmission of STD and possible complications of infection. There is no need to treat the patients partner because avaginitis rarely has serious complications. In men trichomoniasis usually resolves spontaneously.

▼

- Treat for cervicitis and vaginitis
- Educate
- Counsel if needed
- Promote/provide condoms
- Partner management
- Return if necessary

If the patient responds positively to any one of the questions in the decision box for vaginal discharge, treat her for both cervicitis (gonorrhoea and chlamydial infection) and vaginitis (trichomonissis, candidiasis and bacterial vaginosis).

- Treat the patient for voginitis, as above.
- Treat her for cervicitis:

- *For the treatment of gonococcal cervicitis*, give CIPROFLOXACIN 500 mg in a single oral dose, OR CEFTRIAXONE 250 mg single i.m. dose, OR
CEFIXIME 400 mg single oral dose, OR SPECTINOMYCIN 2 9 single i.m. dose.

In regions where kanamycin and cotrimoxazole show continuing efficacy in the treatment of gonorrhoea, these drugs may also be used:
Kanamycin 2 9 single i.m. dose, OR, when single dose therapy is not available:
TRIMETHOPRIM 80 mg/SULPHAMETHOXAZOLE 400 mg (Cotrimoxazole) 10 tablets orally, once a day for three days.

PLUS

- For the treatment of *chlamydial cervicitis,* give DOXYCYCLINE 100 mg orally twice daily for seven days OR
TETRACYCLINE 500 mg orally four times daily for seven days.

Alternatively, the following drugs may be used: ERYTHROMYCIN 500 mg orally four times daily for seven days, OR SULFISOXAZOLE 500 mg orally four times doily for 10 days (equivalent doses of other sulphonumides may also be used)
NOTE: Ciprofloxacin, doxycycline and tetracycline should not be used during pregnancy or lactation.

Before reading further, check with your supervisor which drugs your facility recommends for treating vaginal discharge Make a note of the treatment here:

Now work through the case history below to practise using the flow-chart, then note down what treatment action you will take.

A 25 year old woman complains of a watery discharge. She has had this for two weeks and it is getting worse. She does not know whether or not her partner has a discharge because she has not seen him for two weeks. She has no other symptoms.

Please check your answer with another colleague or your supervisor to make sure that you followed the right pathway through the flow-chart.

E. LOWER ABDOMINAL PAIN

The term pelvic inflammatory disease (PID), refers to infections of the female upper genital tract. It occurs as a result of infection ascending from the cervix and is caused by gonorrhoea, chlamydia and anaerobic bacteria.

PID includes endometritis, salpingitis, tubo-ovarian abscess and pelvic peritonitis. It can also lead to generalized peritonitis, a potentially fatal condition.

In addition, salpingitis may lead to the fallopian tube becoming blocked, resulting in decreased fertility or, if both tubes have become infected, total tubal infertility. It may also lead to partial tubal obstruction, allowing the very small spermatozoa to puss through, but not the larger fertilized ovum. The result can be a tubal pregnancy which will eventually rupture, causing massive intra-abdominal haemorrhoge and, possibly, death.

Women with PID usually present with a history of lower abdominal pain and vaginal discharge. If a woman's symptoms include lower abdominal pain, use the flow-chart below.

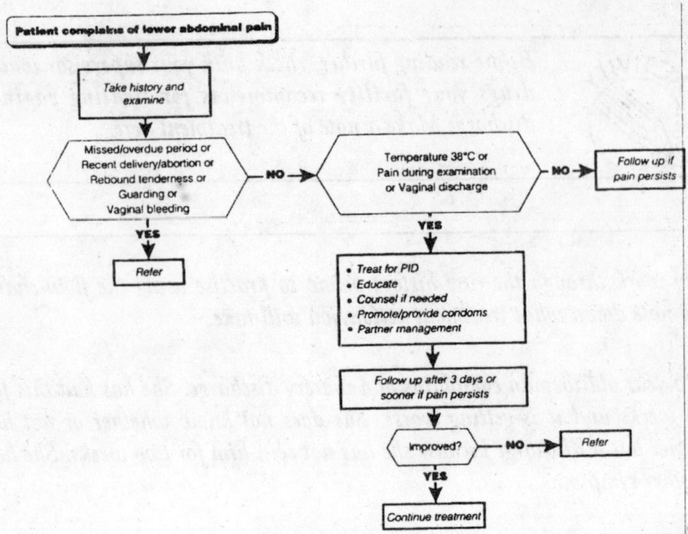

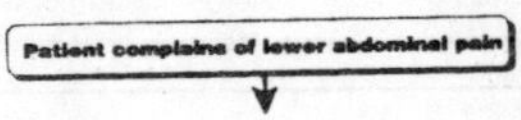

Notice that the entry point to this flow-chart is the symptom of lower abdominal pain. You can also J’ 8 this flow-chart if the patient complains of both lower abdominal pain and vaginal discharge.

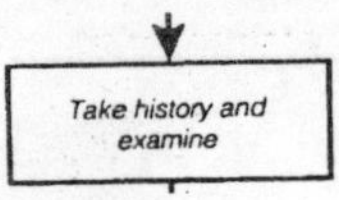

This first action box instructs you to take a history and examine your patient. In the history, you need to check for other symptoms, such a erratic bleeding, missed or overdue period, recent delivery or abortion. Erratic bleeding might be an early symptom of ectopic pregnancy. Ask questions similar to these:

- are there any problems with your periods?
- do you have any vogional bleeding?
- have you hod a miscarriage, abortion or delivery in the last six weeks?

When examining the patient:

1. Check the patient’s temperature. A high temperature indicates infection .
2. Palpate the abdomen for *tenderness, rebound tenderness, guarding* and detection of a *mass.*

   Abdominal palpation should first be superficial to detect pain on light palpation - this is known as tenderness.

   Then make a careful and deep palpation. In the area where you; found tenderness to light palpation, press down slowly and very gently and release the pressure suddenly. Any severe pain that results is known as *rebound tenderness.*

When the peritoneum is inflamed, upon palpation the abdominal muscles will become rigid and will not allow you to apply pressure. This is known as *guarding*. Guarding and rebound tenderness are features of peritonitis or an intra-abdominal abscess.

Light abdominal palpation will also enable you to detect a swelling or lump in the patient's abdomen. This is known as a *moss.* Upon deep palpation of the lower right and lower left abdomen, you might detect a tender mass deep in the pelvic cavity. This may be a tubo-ovarian abscess.

3. See whether the patient has vaginal bleeding. This should alert you to the possibility of an ectopic pregnancy or abortion.
4. See whether the patient has an abnormal vaginal discharged

---

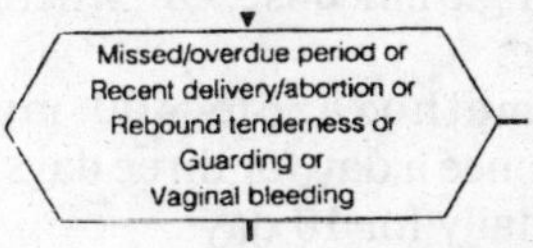

This decision box lists the signs and symptoms for which you must refer the patient. If your examination or the patient's history suggest any of these signs or symptoms, move to the refer box below.

If the patient has none of these signs and symptoms, move to the decision box at next page.

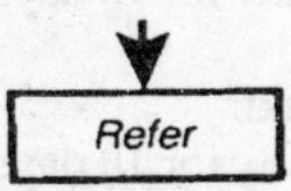

This action box asks you immediately to refer all patients who may have a pregnancy complication, peritonitis or features of tubo-ovarian abscess, as suggested by their symptoms above and/or the signs of rebound tenderness, guarding or your detection of a mass. If so, refer the patient to a facility where specialist gynuecologicol opinion and surgical treatment is available.

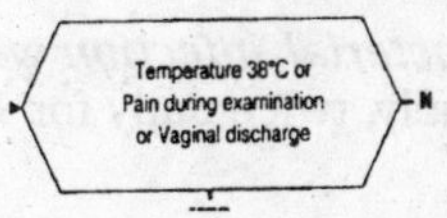

This decision box requires you to make another decision, based on whether or not the patient has a fever of 38° C or more, or tenderness on light palpation, or vaginal discharge.

- If the patient has a fever, pain during examination or a vaginal discharge, treat her for PID as described in the action box below.
- If she has none of these, move to the action box at next page.

Follow up if pain persists

If the patient has none of the warning symptoms and signs in the two decision boxes, reassure the patient and ask her to return if the pain persists .

- Treat for PID
- Educate
- Counsel if needed
- Promote/provide condoms
- Partner management

Remember that, in treating for PID, you must give treatment simultaneously for gonococcal, chlamydial and anaerobic bacterial infection. You must also educate and counsel the patient if necessary, promote and provide condoms, and discuss treating the partner.

- For the treatment for *gonorrhoea,* give
  CIPROFLOXACIN 500 mg in a single oral dose, OR
  CEFTRIAXONE 250 mg single i.m. dose, OR
  CEFIXIME 400 mg single oral dose, OR
  SPECTINOMYCIN 2 9 single i.m. dose.

  In regions where Kanamycin and Cotrimoxazole continue to show efficacy in the treatment of gonorrhoea, these drugs may also be used: Kanamycin 2 g single i.m. dose, OR, where single dose therapy is not available:
  Trimethoprim 80 mg/Sulphomethoxazole 400 mg (Cotrimoxazole) 10 tablets orally, once a day for three days, and then two tablets orally, twice daily for 10 days.

- To treat for *chlamydial infection,* give
  DOXYCYCLINE 100 mg orally, twice daily for 14 days, OR
  TETRACYCLINE 500 mg orally, four times daily for 14 days.

  Alternatively, the following drugs may be used:
  OR Erythromycin 500 mg orally four times daily for 10 days,
  OR Sulfisoxazole 500 mg orally four times daily for 10 days equivalent doses of other *sulphonamides* may also be used).

  NOTE: Ciprofloxacin, doxycycline and tetracycline should not be used during pregnancy or lactation.

- Treat the patient for *anaerobic bacterial infection* with METRONIDAZOLE 400-500 mg orally, twice daily for 1 4 days.

  NOTE: Metronidazole should not be used in the first trimester of pregnancy. Also caution the patient to avoid alcohol while taking this treatment.

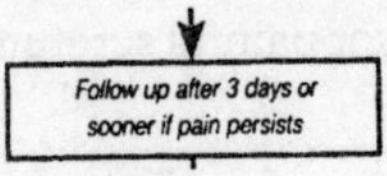

This action box requires that patients should be seen three days after starting treatment, or sooner if pain persists. At this visit, take a history and examine the patient once again.

- If at the follow-up visit the patient is improved, continue the treatment for a total of 10 days.
- If at the follow-up visit the patient is *not* improved, refer her for gynsecological evaluation.

Before reading further check with your supervisor which drugs your facility recommends for treating pelvic inflammatory disease. Make a note of the treatment here:

Now work through the case history below to practise using the flow-chart then note down what treatment action you will take.

A woman's partner has informed her that he has gonorrhoea. She has *no discharge and no fever. She has pain in her left lower abdomen. On palpation, her abdomen is soft, with tenderness on the left side but no guarding. One week later, she returns at your request and is still tender on palpation.*

Please check your answer with another colleague or your supervisor to make sure that you followed the right pathway through the flow-chart.

F. SCROTAL SWELLING

Infection of the testis is a serious complication of gonococcal urethritis and chlamydial urethritis. When infected, the testis becomes swollen, hot and very painful. If early effective therapy is not given, the inflammatory process will resolve and healing occurs with fibrous scarring and destruction of testicular tissue. This will decrease the patient's fertility.

Patients who complain of having a swollen and/or painful scrotum may be managed by using this flow-chart.

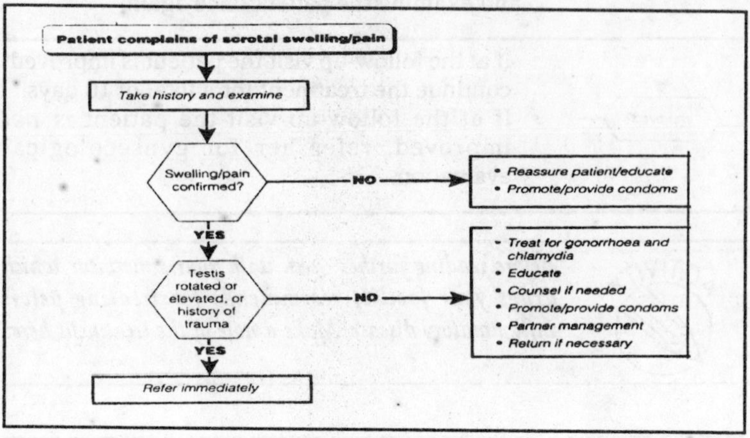

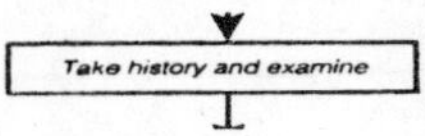

This first action box advises you to take a history and examine the patient. In the history, note these two points:

1. Has the patient injured himself?
2. Has the patient hod an STD in the last six weeks?

On examining the patient, note these six points:

1. Palpate the scrotal sac comparing the two sides. Is there swelling of the testis? Is there pain in the testis?
2. What is the position of the testis in the scrotal sac? Is it elevated or rotated? If so, this is known as torsion.
3. Is there bruising of the scrotal skin which could indicate trauma?
4. Is there an obvious urethral discharge? If not, ask the patient to squeeze the penis and milk the urethra in order to express any discharge.
5. Is there evidence of any other STD?
6. Is there swelling in the inguinal area or does the scrotal swelling increase when the patient raises the intra-abdominal pressure (straining as if passing stools)? This may point to an inguinal hernia and requires referral to a surgical facility.

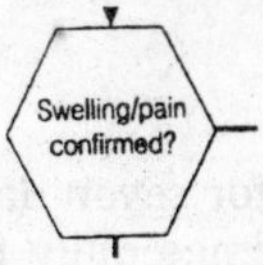

This decision box asks whether or not the swelling or pain is confirmed.

- If you have no positive findings after taking the patient's history and examining him, the swelling is not confirmed. Follow the instructions in the 'Reassure patient' action box to the right: explain that you can find no signs of swelling, educate him on safer sex, promote the use of condoms and ask him to return if symptoms persist.
- If you can confirm the presence of swelling and/or pain in the testis, move to the action box below.

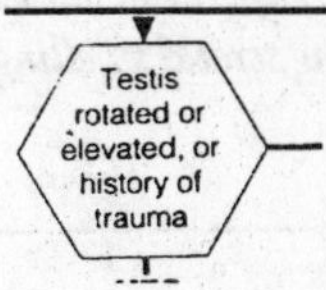

If the patient has swelling and/or pain in the scrotum, this decision box asks you to check whether the testis is elevated or retested.

- If this is so, refer the patient to a facility where a surgical or urological opinion can be obtained.
- If there is a history of trauma, refer the patient.
- If you think the patient has a scrotal hernia after examining him, refer him to a surgical facility (see 6 above).
- If none of the above factors can apply to the swelling or pain, treat the patient as described in the action box to the right.

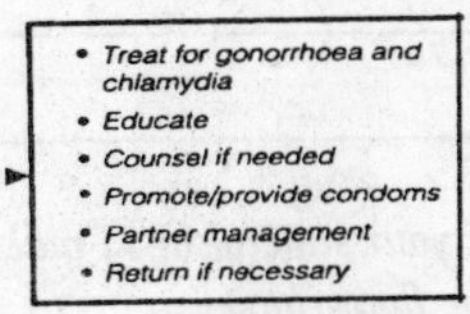

This action box asks you to treat the patient for gonorrhoea and chlamydia, and also to educate the patient and counsel him If needed, promote safe sex and condom use, manage sexual partners and ask the patient to return if symptoms persist.

- Treat the patient for gonorrhoea and chlamydial infection as follows:
- for the treatment of gonococcal urethritis, give CIPROFLOXACIN 500 mg in a single oral dose, OR CEFTRIAXONE 250 mg single i.m. dose, OR CEFIXIME 400 mg single oral dose, OR SPECTINOMYCIN 2g single i.m. dose.

In regions where *kanamycin* and *cotrimoxazole* show continuing efficacy in the treatment of gonorrhoea, these drugs may also be used:
Kanomycin 2 g single i.m. dose, OR, when single dose therapy is not available:
Trimethoprim 80 mg/Sulphomethoxazole 400 mg (Cotrimoxazole) 10 tablets orally, once a day for three days.

PLUS

- For *chlamydial urethritis,* give DOXYCYCLINE 100 mg orally twice daily for seven days OR TETRACYCLINE 500 mg orally four times daily for seven days.

  Alternatively, the following drugs may be used: *Erythromycin* 500 mg orally four times daily for seven days, OR *Sulfisoxazole* 500 mg orally four times doily for 10 days (equivalent doses of other *sulphonamides* may also be used)

Before reading further, check with your supervisor which drugs your facility recommends for treating scrotal swelling. Make a note of the treatment here:

Now work through the case history below to practise using the flow-chart, then note down what treatment action you will take.

A young man comes into the clinic complaining of a painful groin. The testes are swollen and painful, with no history or evidence of trauma or torsion.

Please check your answer with another colleague or your supervisor to make sure that you followed the right pathway through the flow-chart.

G. INGUINAL BUBO

This is a painful, often fluctuant, swelling of the Iymph nodes in the inguinal region lgroin). Buboes are usually coused by either chancroid or lymphogrunuloma venereum (LGV).

When LGV is the cause, there is usually no ulcer present. On the other hand, a bubo and an ulcer suggest that the patient has chancroid, so you must refer to the genital ulcer flow-chart and treat him/her for these.

If a patient complains of having a painful inguinal swelling (bubo), use this flowchart:

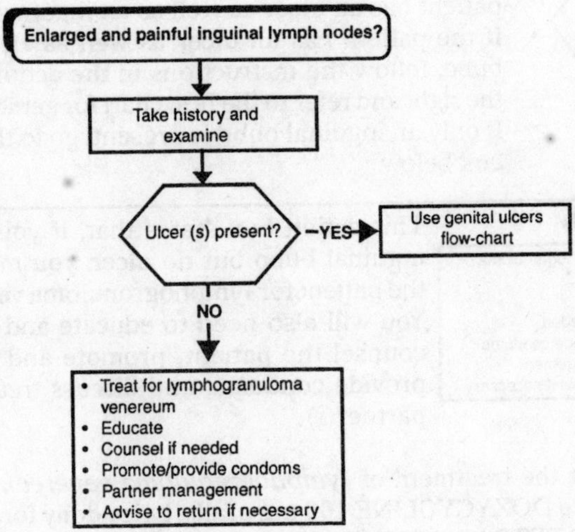

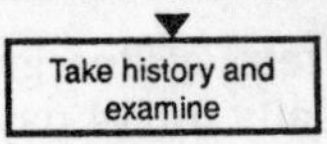

This action box requires you to take a history and examine the patient. When you take the history, ask:

1. Is there pain in the groin?
2. Do you also have a genital ulcer, or have you recently had a genital ulcer?
3. Have you noticed any swellings elsewhere in the body?

When examining the patient, try and determine whether the swelling is really a bubo or simply enlarged lymph nodes or any other pathology which has enlarged nodes in other sites. A bubo is usually painful, warm, tender to palpation and fluctuant. There may be one large mass or a collection of smaller painful swellings. Occasionally the bubo might have ruptured and a sinus discharging pus will be present

If a bubo is present, make sure to look for genital ulcers:

- in men, remember to examine the underside of the foreskin and the parts normally covered by the foreskin. If the patient cannot retract the foreskin because of swelling, assume there is a genital ulcer and use the appropriate flow-chart;
- in women, examine the skin of the external genitulia and then separate the lobia and look at the mucous surface for ulcers.

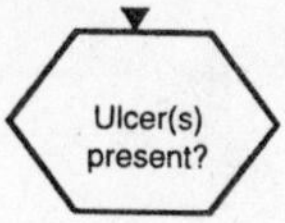

This decision box asks you whether or not the patient has an ulcer as well as an inguinal bubo.

- If the patient has an ulcer as well as an inguinal bubo, follow the instructions in the action box on the right and refer to the flowchart for genital ulcers.
- If only an inguinal bubo is present, go to the action box below.

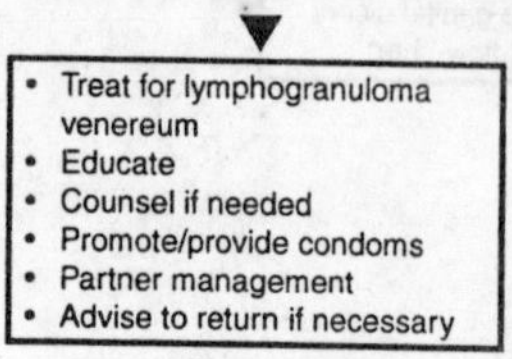

This action box states that, if you find an inguinal bubo but no ulcer, you must treat the patient for Iymphogronuloma venereum. You will also need to educate and perhaps counsel the patient, promote and perhaps provide condoms, and discuss treating the partner(s).

- For the treatment of *Iymphogranuloma venereum* {LGV), give DOXYCYCLINE 100 mg orally, twice doily for 14 days, OR TETRACIACLINE 500 mg orally, four times daily for 14 days.

  Alternatively, for those who cannot tolerate tetracycline, give Erythromycin 500 mg orally, four times daily for 14 days, OR *Sulfadiazine* 1 g orally, four times doily for 14 days.

  NOTE: Tetracycline should not be used during pregnancy and lactation.

  If a bubo becomes fluctuant, pus should be aspirated with a needle through the adjeet healthy skin. Repeat aspiration after two to three days if necessary. Never incise a bubo.

ACTIVITY

Before reading further, check with your supervisor which drugs your facility recommends for treating inguinal bubo. Make a note of the treatment here: .

____

____

____

Now work through the case history below to practise using the flow-chart, then note down what treatment action you will take.

A young man attends the clinic because of severe pain in the groin. He has had several different sexual partners over the last few months and does not use condoms on a regular basis. There is no visible sore on the penis, but there is a large, swollen node in the right groin.

____

____

____

Please check your answer with another colleague or your supervisor to make sure that you followed the right pathway through the flow-chart.

H. NEONATAL CONJUNCTIVITIS

Ophthalmia neonatorum is defined as purulent conjunctivitis occurring in a baby less than one month of age. The common causes of this potentially sight-threatening condition are *gonorrhoea* and *chlamydia*. If the baby is older, the cause is unlikely to be an STD.

Prevention of ophthalmia neonatorum

All newly born babies should have *preventive* therapy carried out as follows:

- as soon as the baby is born, wipe both eyes with dry, clean cotton wool;
- then apply 1% tetracycline eye ointment into the lower conjunctival sacs of both eyes;
- remember that the baby's eyes are usually swollen soon after birth and may be difficult to open. Therefore, the eyes should be opened and the eye ointment placed in the lower conjunctival sacs and not on the eyelids.

Management of ophthalmia neonatorum

If a baby of less than one month has swollen eyes and pus, use the flow-chart on the next page.

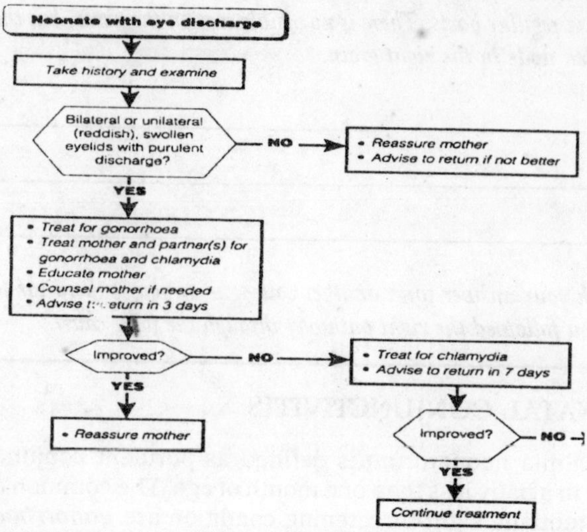

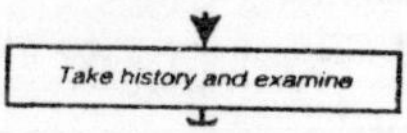

This first action box tells you to take a history from the mother and examine the baby. Ask the mother if she or her sexual partner(s) have any STD symptoms.

Examine the baby, looking specifically for a purulent conjunctival discharge. The baby's eyes are usually closed, and the eyelids swollen. You will notice that, when the eyelids are separated or pressed, pus pours out from beneath them.

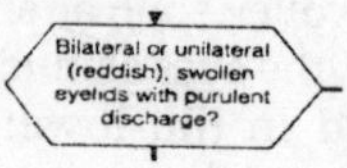

If one or both eyes are swollen with a purulent discharge, move to the action box below.

If purulent can junctivitis is not found, move to the action box or the right, which asks you to reassure the mother and ask her to return with the baby if symptoms persist.

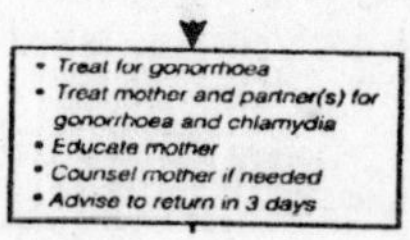

This action box requires that, if purulent conjunctivitis is present, you treat the baby for gonorrhoea and the mother and partner for both gonorrhoea and chlamydia. Notice that, at this point, the baby receives treatment only for the one condition; treatment for chlamydia will follow only if the baby's eyes do not improve. Remember to also educate and treat the mother and partners).

- FOR THE BABY, the treatment for *gonococcal ophthalmia is:*
  - CEFTRIAXONE 50 mg/kg (maximum 125 mg) in a single i.m. dose.

Where ceftriaxone is not available, use:
Kanamycin 25 mg/kg (maximum 75 mg) in a single i.m. dose, OR Spectinomycin 25 mg/kg (maximum 75 mg) in a single i.m. dose.
Clean the *baby's eyes with saline or clean* water, *using a* clean *swab for each eye. Remember to* clean *from* the inside to the *outside edge of each eye. Wash your hands carefully afterwards.*

- The MOTHER and the MOTHER'S PARTNER(S) should be given treatment for *gonorrhoea and chlamydial infection.*
  - For *gonorrhoea,* give
    CEFTRIAXONE 250 mg single i.m. dose, OR
    SPECTINOMYCIN 2 g single i.m. dose, OR
    CEFIXIME 400 mg single oral dose, OR
    CIPROFLOXACIN 500 mg in a single oral dose.

    If the above therapies are not available, give Kanamycin 2g single i.m. dose, OR,
    if single dose therapy is not available: Trimethoprim 80 mg/ Sulphamethoxazole 400 mg (Cotrimoxazole) 10 tablets orally, once a day for three days.

  PLUS

  - For *chlamydial infection,* give
    DOXYCYCLINE 100 mg orally, twice daily for seven days, OR
    TETRACYCLINE 500 mg orally, four times daily for seven days.
    Where tetracyclines are not advised, give:
    Erythromycin 500 mg orally, four times daily for seven days, OR
    Sulfafurazole 500 mg orally, four times daily for 10 days (equivalent doses of other sulphonumides may also be used).

    NOTE: Ciprofloxacin, doxycycline and tetracycline should not be used by lactating women.

- Advise the mother to complete the course of tablets and educate her about the mode of transmission of STD, the nature of the baby's infection, how to clean the baby's eyes and possible complications of infection. Counsel her if necessary and promote the use of condoms.
- Ask the mother to return for follow-up in three days if that is convenient to her, and stress that she must return if the symptoms in either her or the baby persist.

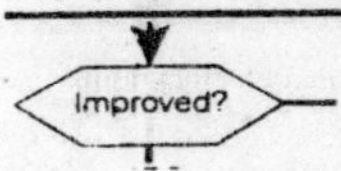

Upon the patients' return, preferably within 72 hours, this decision box requires that you examine the baby. If the discharge has improved, reassure the mother and remember to reinforce the education message. If it has not improved, move to the action box at next page.

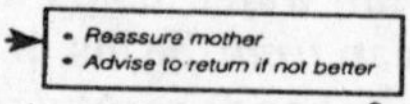

If the baby's eyes are still discharging pus:

- Treat the baby for *chlamydial infection* with ERYTHROMYCIN SYRUP 50 mg/kg/day orally four times daily for 14 days.

Alternatively, give:
Trimethoprim 40 mg/Sulphamethoxazole 200 mg orally twice daily for 14 days.

- Ask the mother to return with the baby in seven days.

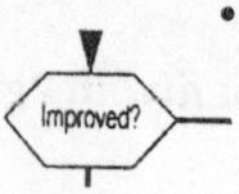

- If the baby is improved at the second follow-up visit, move to the action box below. No further treatment is necessary but, as the box indicates, you must urge the mother to complete the 14 days' treatment. Reinforce education and counselling messages.
- If on the second follow-up visit symptoms persist (despite treatment for gonococcal and chlamydial ophthalmia neonotorum) move to the action box on the right, which states that you should refer the baby for poediatric or ophthalmic

---

Before reading further, check with your supervisor which drugs your facility recommends for treating neonatal conjunctivitis. Make a note of the treatment here:

Now work through the case history below to practise using the flow-chart, then note down what treatment action you will take.

A two-week old baby is brought into the clinic with an obvious eye infection. One eye appears swollen, the other is swollen and discharging yellow pus.

The mother brings the baby back after the weekend complaining that the eye infection is no better.

Please check your answer with another colleague or your supervisor to make sure that you followed the right pathway through the flow-chart.

I. REVIEW

In this workbook, you have read all the guidance on syndromic diagnosis and treatment of STD.

The workbook contains lots of detail, so you now need time to digest what you have read, and to begin to apply it.

To help you with this important aspect of your learning, the remaining pages contain questions (as well as the answers!) and an action plan.

The aim of the questions is to help you understand and remember specific details in the flow-charts. It is a chance to check your learning and practise applying it in some small case studies.

Please take your time over the questions, and check your answers carefully with ours. Feel free to refer back to specific flow-charts and their associated text at any time.

The action plan contains some suggestions on how you make the flow-charts as accessible as possible at your place of work.

Finally, please use the space below to note down any questions or concerns you have about anything in this workbook, and be sure to discuss them soon with your tutor or supervisor.

My questions and concerns

J. SELF-CHECK QUESTIONS

1. *When is a vaginal discharge NOT a problem?*

2. *Here are three questions about assessing risk factors:*

a) *For what syndrome is it useful to assess risk factors?*

b) *In assessing a patient's risk we need to take four factors into account. What are they?*

c) *What two extra questions must you ask in addition to the risk factors?*

3. *When a patient complains of scrotal swelling:*

   a) *What two questions must you add when taking the patients history?*

   b) *While examining the patient who complains of scrotal swelling, what six signs should you look for particularly?*

4. *How does an inguinal bubo differ from an enlarged inguinal lymph node?*

5. *On the next few pages are seven short case studies. For each one, please decide what flow-chart you would use, then read what happens when you take the patient's history and examine him or her. We will then ask you how to treat the patient.*

   a) *Mas is a young boy of 15 years who lives in the slum area of Diredawa. He has been brought to the district hospital because his scrotum is swollen and he is vomiting. What flowchart do you use?*

___

___

___

On examination, the scrotum is swollen and painful; the testes elevated and rotated. How do you manage this patient?

___

___

___

b) *Gloria took her four-day old baby to the clinic when she noticed that his right eye was swollen and there was pus in both eyes (the right eye more than the left). What flow-chart do you use?*

___

___

What treatment do you offer, to whom?

c) *Donna, aged 22, attended the family planning clinic for her usual check-up while on the contraceptive pill. She tells the nurse about a yellow, itchy vaginal discharge that she has had for the past four days. What flow-chart do you use?*

___

___

Donna says she has no abdominal pain or dysuria. She had her menses two weeks ago and it was normal. Shyly, she discloses that she had sex with an old school friend a week ago, and that she did not use a condom because she was on the pill. She last had sex with her regular boyfriend a month ago, as he was out of town. For what do you treat Donna?

---

d) *An 18 year old dock worker attends your clinic complaining that he had a discharge yesterday. What flow-chart do you use?*

On examination, you can find no discharge, even after milking the urethra. However you do find an ulcer on his penis. What do you do now?

For what do you treat this patient?

---

e) *24 year-old Anne states that she began seeing Tom, her new partner, three months ago. She is now experiencing a dull 'persistent belly bottom pain which she thinks has been brought on by her excessive sexual activity with Tom. What flow-chart do you use?*

Anne tells you that her periods are normal and she has never been pregnant. She thought that there might be some increase in what she considers to be normal vaginal discharge. On examination, she has no rebound tenderness or guarding, but clearly feels pain when you palpate the lower abdomen. What treatment do you give to Anne?

What else do you discuss with her?

---

f) *Richard says he noticed a slight pain in his left groin. Two days later, he noticed that it looked swollen. He has rushed to the clinic after work. What flow-chart do you use?*

On examination, you find that he has a small sore on his penis. His left groin is tender and swollen. What treatment do you offer Richard?

---

6. *Finally, below are four case studies to give you more practice in diagnosing the cause or causes of vaginal discharge. Please decide whether you need to treat each woman for vaginitis only, or for both vaginitis and cervicitis.*

---

a) *Sarah moved in with her present partner four months ago. She is 22. In addition to the discharge, she says her lower abdomen feels tender. Her partner has no symptoms.*

---

b) *Jasmin complains of a slight vaginal discharge. She is 25 years old and has been married for eight years. Her third child was born four months ago, so she's been busy caring for him at home. Apart from this discharge, she feels well and has no other symptoms.*

---

c) *Ami is a 17 year old in an urban area in Africa. She reports a slight discharge but no other symptoms. She has lived with her current boyfriend for nine months.*

---

d) *34 year-old Sharma complains of a slight yellow discharge. She has not been with anyone since her husband left home six months ago. She has no other symptoms.*

K. ACTION PLAN

Below we suggest some ways you can practise syndromic diagnosis using the flow-charts. Please adopt them according to what you most need to learn or practise, given your prior experience and learning.

Check what drugs are available and effective for each condition

This is an important priority so, if you have not done so already, find out what drugs are available to treat each syndrome. At the buck of the workbook, you will find a special page to record locally recommended drugs.

Make sure you have easy access to a list of the locally recommended drugs. You might, for example, write them on a piece of paper or curd that you could keep on your desk, or note them on each flow-chart if you have quick-reference copies or a large wall-chart of them.

Confirm the risk factors that you will use

The risk factors used for vaginal discharge syndrome were developed for Africa. For countries elsewhere they may need to be amended. Please consult your tutor or supervisor on this matter if you haven't already done so.

Practise using the flow-charts

- act you arrange to practise using the flow-charts with colleagues?
- act out managing different syndromes in pairs, remembering to ask the appropriate questions and include the necessary advice;
- a third person could observe you both, with the workbook open at the appropriate pages to check that you do not miss out anything,
- it you do not have colleagues to work with, imagine a patient and work through what you would ask and do with the appropriate flow-chart open but the workbook closed. You could then read through the workbook to check how you have done.

As soon as you feel confident about using the flow-charts, arrange to practice syndromic diagnosis and treatment at your local health centre.

L. ANSWERS

If you are a clinician or have already worked with STD, you may have found these questions very easy. On the other hand, if all this is new, it will take longer to reach the point where you feel confident about syndromic diagnosis - so don't worry if you found the questions difficult. Remember their purpose is to help you learn.

1. Vaginal discharge is physiological or normal both during and after sexual activity, be^fore, during and after a menstrual period, and during pregnancy and location. Remember that most women will not seek medical attention unless they perceive the discharge to be different or unusual in some way
2. a) An assessment of specific risk factors is mode for vaginal discharge. Remember that the purpose is to decide whether the discharge is coused by vaginitis alone or by both voginitis and cervicitis.

   b) In assessing a patient's risk we need to take four factors into account On the African continent, these are the four factors:
      1. Less than 21 years of age.
      2. Single.
      3. More than one partner in the last three months.
      4. A new partner in the last three months.

   c) In addition to the risk factors, you must also ask:
      - is the patient's partner symptomatic?
      - does the patient have pain in the lower abdomen?

      Remember that the patient should be treated for both cervicitis as well as vaginitis if one or more of these two questions or of the four risk factors is answered positively.
3. a) When interviewing a patient who complains of scrotal swelling, these are the two questions to ask:
      - has he injured himself?
      - has he had an STD in the last six weeks?

   b) This was quite a difficult question, so very good if you remembered all six of the signs to look for during the examination:
      - swelling or pain in the testis when you palpate the scrotal sac;
      - testis elevated or rotated;
      - bruising of the scrotal skin;
      - an obvious urethral discharge;
      - evidence of any other STD;
      - evidence of an inguinal hernia.

Remember that you can check for inguinal hernia by asking the patient to raise the intra-abdominal pressure.

4. An inguinal bubo differs from an enlarged inguinal lymph node in that it is usually painful, warm, tender to palpation and fluctuation. We also stressed that it can take the form of either one large mass or a collection of smaller swellings, and that occasionally it might rupture, so that you will see a sinus discharging pus.

5. a) The correct flow-chart to use for this patient is the one for scrotal swelling, .

   The management guidelines state that you should refer Mas immediately. He might have a torsion of his testicles.

   b) The correct syndrome and flow-chart to use for Gloria's baby is the one for neonatal conjunctivitis.

   We hope you noticed that, while at first the baby is treated only for gonorrhoea (gonococcal ophthalmia), the mother and her partner(s) must be treated for both gonorrhoea and chlamydia. An important feature of this flow-chart is that the baby is only treated for chlamydial infection if there is no improvement after taking the initial treatment for gonorrhoea.

   c) The correct flow-chart to use for Diona is vaginal discharge. Well done if you wrote that Donna should be treated for both cervicitis and vaginitis. Why? Because she has had sex with more than one person in the last three months, which is one of the risk factors to take into account. She might also be positive on a second risk factor - sex with a new partner in the last three months. However, we can't be sure whether or not the 'old school friend' is a new sexual partner and in any case only one positive risk factor is sufficient to treat Donna for both causes.

   d) You are quite right to select the flow-chart for urethral discharge at first, because this is the symptom of which the patient complains.

   Given the result of your examination, the flow-chart redirects you to the one for *genital ulcer.*

   Examination has already confirmed that the patient has an ulcer so you must treat him for both syphilis and chancroid.

   e) The correct flow-chart to use given Anne's symptoms is the one for lower abdominal pain.

   Upon examination, the pain in Anne's lower abdomen suggests that she has pelvic inflammatory disease. She should be treated for gonorrhoea, chlamydia *and* anaerobic bacterial infection. The treatment WHO recommends for these is:

Gonorrhoea -	Ciprofloxacin 500 mg in a single oral dose.
Chlamydia -	Doxycycline 100 mg orally twice daily for 14 days.
Anaerobic bacterial infection -	Metronidazole 400-500 mg orally twice daily for 14 days.

Please remember that pain during examination is not the only decisive sign. Either an observed vaginal discharge or a temperature of 38°C, in addition to her given symptom of lower abdominal pain, would have been sufficient to lead to a diagnosis of PID.

The action box also lists the other important aspects of comprehensive case management of STD.

f) The correct initial flow-chart for Richard's symptom is the one for inguinal bubo.

Upon examination you confirm that Richard's groin is both swollen and tender. This is a sign of inguinal bubo. However the patient has an ulcer, so the flow-chart and text stress that you must use the flow-chart for genital ulcers - well done if you mode this decision. The treatment to offer Richard is therefore for chancroid. Notice that the drug treatment for these causes would also be effective if the cause was lymphogronuloma venereum. If the swelling shows signs of fluid retention, you also need to aspirate the bubo.

6. In deciding whether to treat a woman with vaginal discharge for one or two causative agents, only one of the factors or questions need be positive. So how did you do with the four examples? (By the way, we assume that you are using the risk factors identified in the workbook. If you have already been given different factors, please check your answers with your tutor or supervisor.)
   a) Sarah says that lower abdominal pain is one of her symptoms - so she needs treatment for both cervicitis and voginitis.
   b) Jasmin's case is more difficult. The information we have given suggests that she needs to be treated only for vaginitis because the risk factors are negative. But we haven't asked if her partner has any symptoms. To be sure of the appropriate treatment, we would need to check all the risk factors first.
   c) As to Ami, we know that she is less than 21 years old. This is one of the four risk factors, so we hope that you decided to treat her for both voginitis and cervicitis.

d) Sharma is the only person we can confidently treat for vaginitis alone because none of the risk factors or questions apply in her case.

GLOSSARY

Action box The rectangular box on a flow-chart that tells you to do something, for example, take history, treat or educate

Anaerobic bacteria Bacteria that grow without air or need an oxygenfree environment to live, usually Bacteriodes species, one of the causes of PID

Aspirste Draw fluid away by suction e.g. draw pus out of an *inguinal bubo*

Candidiasis Condition coused by the yeastlike fungus *Candida albicans* (also known as 'thrush') that is one of the causes of *voginitis*

Cerervscitis Inflammation of the *cervix*, usually caused by *gonorrhoea* or chlamydia

Cervix The neck of the uterus (womb)

Chancroid STD caused by the bacterium Haemophilus ducreyi

Chlomydia Infection with the bacterium *Chlamydium trachomatis;* one of the causes of vaginal and urethral discharge, and of discharging eyes if newborns

Complications Secondary diseases or conditions that can arise if a disease is not treated

Decision box The six-sided box on a flow-chart that asks you to obtain information and make a decision

Dysuria Painful or difficult urination

Ectopic pregnancy A potentially fatal condition caused by a pregnancy that occurs outside the uterus (usually in the fallopian tubes)

Efficacy The measure of how effective a treatment is

Endometritis Inflammation of the endometrium (lining of the uterus)

Fibrous scarring Scarring that looks like or consists of, fibres

Fluctuant/ Fluctuation Description of fluid that moves to and fro, as does pus within a bubo

Genital ulcer disease The name for the *syndrome* where ulcers or sores are found in the genital region, usually caused by *syphilis* and chancroid

Gonorrhoea/ gonorrhea STD caused by the bacterium *Neisseria* gonorrhoeae

Gonococcal Caused by gonorrhoea, as in *gonococcal urethritis*

Guarding During examination of women for the syndrome

	lower abdominal pain you may find that the abdominal muscles become rigid and do not allow you to apply pressure - this is known as guarding. is usually a sign of *peritonitis* or an intra *abdominal abscess* - both potentially serious conditions
Gynaecological	Concerning the physiological functions and diseases of the female reproductive system
Herpes	STD coused by the *Herpes simplex virus (HSV)*
i; m	Abbreviation for 'intra-muscularly' meaning into or within muscle
Inguinal bubo(es)	Name of the *syndrome* where the patient complains of a painful swelling of the lymph nodes in the groin, usually caused by *LGV*
Inguinal hernia	A ruptured muscle wall in the groin through which internal organs may be partly displaced
Intra-abdominal abscess	A potentially serious abscess inside the abdomina cavity
Intravaginally	Into or within the vagina
Lactation	Another term for breast-feeding
LGV	An abbreviation for the *STD* lymphogronuloma venereum, caused by *Chlamydia trachomatis*
Lower abdominal pain	The name for the *syndrome* where women complain of pain in the lower abdomen, which is usually - but not always - coused by *pelvic inflammatory disease* (PID)
Lymphogranuloma venereum	STD caused by the bacterium *Chlamydia trachomatis* which can lead to the *syndrome of inguinal bubo* and also *lower abdominal* pain
Mass	Lump of tissue (often malignant)
Mucous membrane	Mucous-secreting tissue lining many body cavities and tubular organs
Neisseria gonorrhoeae	Scientific name for the bacterium which causes gonorrhoea
Neonatal conjunctivitis	Inflammation of the mucous membranes of the eyes or eyelids as a result of *gonorrhoea* or *chlamydia* spreading to a baby's eyes as it passes through the *cervix* and vagina during birth
Ophthalmia neonatorum	*Conjunctivitis* occurring in a baby less than one month old, usually due to gonorrhoea or chlamydial infection
Ophthalmic	Concerning the physiological functions and diseases of the eyes
Oral dose	Drugs taken by mouth

Ovum/ova	Fertilised egg or eggs (ova is plural)
Paediatric	Concerning the physiological functions and diseases of children
Palpate/palpation	To examine by touch
Pelvic inflammatory disease	One of the causes of the syndrome *lower abdominal pain,* which is in turn caused by *gonorrhoea, chlamydia* and/or *anaerobic bacteria*
Peritoneum	Lining of the abdominal cavity
Peritonitis	Inflammation of the peritoneum
Physiological	Healthy/normal functioning
PID	An abbreviation for *pelvic inflammatory disease,* one of the causes of the syndrome lower abdominal pain
Prenatal	Of or relating to, the time before childbirth
Purulent	Discharging pus
Rebound tenderness	This is one of the signs of peritonitis or an *intra abdominal abscess* which you would look for during an examination for the syndrome *lower abdominal pain.* The patient will feel severe pain when you press down slowly and gently on a tender area and then suddenly release the pressure. Along with *guarding* it is usually a sign of potentially serious condition(s).
Salpingitis	Inflammation of the *fallopian tubes*
Scrotal swelling	The name for the *syndrome* where men present with a swollen, hot and painful *testis/testes,* usually but not always as a result of infection by *gonorrhoea* or chlamydia
Sign	A clinical problem you can see by examination, together with *symptom(s)* making a *syndrome*
Sinus	A tube or passage to an *abscess*
Spermatozoa	Mature motile sperm cells
STD	An abbreviation for sexually transmitted disease(s)
Syndrome	A collection of *symptoms* and signs
Syphilis	STD coused by the bacterium *Treponema palladium*
Symptom	a clinical problem which the patient complains of, together with sign(s) making a *syndrome*
Symptomatic	Showing characteristic symptoms
Testis	The medical *name* for *a testicle (plural is* testes)
Trauma	*Any* physical wound or injury, sometimes also used *to* describe the shock following a wound *or injury*
Trichomonas vaginalis	Scientific name for the bacterium that causes *the* STD trichomoniosis
Trichomoniasis	STD caused *by the* bacterium *Trichomonas* vaginalis
Tubal	*A* potentially fatal pregnancy that occurs in *the*

pregnancy	fallopian tubes
Tubo-ovarian abscess	*A* potentially serious abscess in *the fallopian* tubes or ovaries
Unilateral	Affecting only one eye (of *conjunctivitis)*
Urological	Of *the* urinary *system*
Uterine cavity	Body *cavity containing the uterus*
Urethra	*The duct* by which urine is discharged from *the* bladder (see *also urethritis)*
Urethral	*The name* of *the syndrome* where *the patient* presents *with a discharge from the urethra,* usually caused by *gonorrhoea or* chlamydia
Urethritis	Inflammation of *the urethra,* usually caused by *gonorrhoea or* chlamydia
Vaginal bacteriosis	Another term for *bacterial vaginosis, the* organism *Gardnerella vaginalis which is one of the causes* of *vaginitis*
Vaginal discharge	*The name* of *the syndrome* where *the patient presents with a discharge from the* vagina, usually caused by *gonorrhoea or* chlamydia
Vaginitis	*Inflammation of the* vagina caused by *bacterial* vaginosis/vaginal bacteriosis, *trichomoniosis or* candidiasis
Vesicular lesions	*Rash of* tiny blisters before *they burst and form a* sore, caused by the Herpes simplex virus (HSV)

DRUG TREATMENTS

Urethral Discharge

Gonococcal urethritis Treatment: ____________________

____

____

plus ____________________

Notes: ____________________

Chlamydial urethritis Treatment: ____________________

____

____

____

Notes: ____________________

Genital Ulcers
Syphilis Treatment: ____________________

____

____

plus ____________________

Notes: ____________________

Chancroid — Treatment: ______

______

______

Notes: ______

Vaginal Discharge

Risk assessment negative:
Treat for Vaginitis: Treatment: ______
Trichomoniasis, ______
Bacterial vaginosis ______
plus ______
Vaginal candidissis, Notes: ______

Risk assessment positive:
Treat for Vaginitis *Treatment:* ______
(as above}: ______

______

plus Notes: ______

Treat for Cervicitis Treatment: ______

______

______

______

Notes: ______

Lower Abdominal Pain

Gonorrhoea Treatment: ______

______

plus ______

______

Notes: ______

Chlumydia Treatment: ______

plus ______

______

______

Notes: ______

Anaerobic bacterial infection Treatment: ______

______

______

______

Notes: ______

Scrotal Swelling

Gonococcul urethritis — Treatment: ____________________

plus

Notes: ____________________

Chlamydisl urethritis — Treatment: ____________________

Notes: ____________________

Inguinal Bubo

Lymphogrunuloma venereum — Treatment: ____________________

Notes: ____________________

Neonatal Conjunctivitis

Treat baby for Gonococcal ophthalmia — Treatment: ____________________

Notes: ____________________

If no improvement within 72 hours, treat for Chlamydial infection — Treatment: ____________________

Notes: ____________________

Treat mother and partner(s) for Gonorrhoea — Treatment: ____________________

plus

Notes: ____________________

For Chlamydial infection — Treatment: ____________________

Notes: ____________________

6

EDUCATING THE PATIENT

A. INTRODUCTION

Welcome to this, the fifth workbook in STD case management.

The subject of this workbook is educating the patient and motivating him or her to change their sexual behaviour - as you know, a challenging objective!

Education is the third of the five steps in STD case management. It follows the first two steps: history taking and examination, and making a syndromic diagnosis.

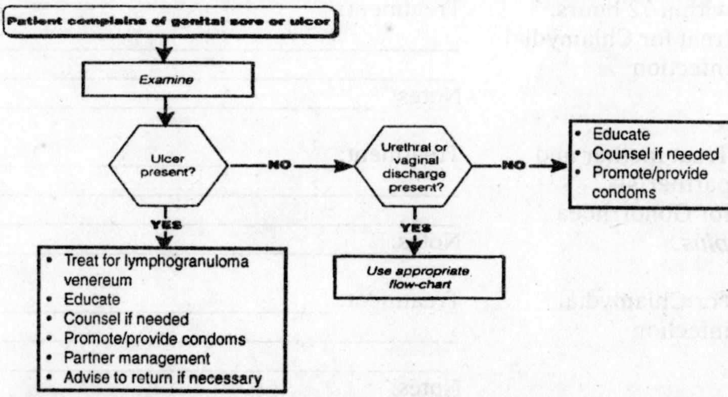

The goals of educating a patient with STD are to help the patient resolve the current infection and prevent future ones.

In Workbook 3, we stressed that the purpose of history taking was both to obtain accurate information as *efficiently* as possible and to gain the patient's confidence. Once you have diagnosed an STD, you need to add three further aims:

- to educate the patient on a number of issues;
- to motivate the patient to adopt behaviours that resolve the current infection and prevent future ones;
- to provide the patient with emotional support.

The interviewing skills we explored in Workbook 3 are also essential for this part of the interview. You might like to use the questions below to help you recall those skills.

QUESTION

1. Can you remember the interviewing skills we covered in Workbook 3? Try answering these two questions:

a) We mentioned two types of question: what are they?

Which type of question is it best to use when taking the patient's history? Why?

b) What are the six verbal skills we suggested? Note down as many as you can recall!

Why is patient education important?

Health centres and clinics are often very busy places. Nevertheless, we have stressed the importance of using every opportunity to educate patients with STD. Why? And why should it happen at the health centre?

- clinic-based education is efficient because it reaches people where they already are: the patient has come to you;
- the clinic visit is a unique opportunity for patient education. Often the only time that patients are interested to learn about a disease or its prevention is once they, or someone they know, are faced with that disease. Therefore, clinics offering education do so at the *right moment for the patient to learn,*
- treatment is more effective if patients understand their illness and why they should comply with treatment. There will be less morbidity due to STDs.

- STDs can recur; preventing them requires sustained behaviour change. While patients might be willing to comply with treatment for a current infection, they often need education, motivation and emotional support to adopt practices that will prevent a recurrence of STD.
- by increasing the frequency of patient compliance with treatment and behaviour change, education also helps to prevent future infection by either STD or HIV.

Your learning objectives

By the end of this workbook, you will be able to:

- explain why educating and motivating patients is so vital in managing STD cases;
- identify the main topics on which to educate STD patients;
- recognise and practise a number of additional skills during this part of the interview;
- demonstrate the use of condoms.

The workbook contains action plans to help you to practise these steps and skills.

B. EDUCATE ON WHAT?

This section will enable you to identify a number of issues on which you need to educate STD patients.

As with any patient, all those with an STD need to know about their medication: when to take it and for how long, the importance of completing the medication even if the patient feels better, and so on. With STD patients there are also many other issues to explain and discuss.

We could simply tell you what these issues are, but try working them out for yourself first, by answering this question.

QUESTION

2. *In educating patients with STD, what issues do you need to discuss or explore with them? In answering this question, you might find it helpful to refer to the flow-charts.*

Our answer to question 2 is a summary of the main issues to discuss with an STD patient. We have listed them in the order in which you would most likely discuss them. Here are the points once again:

1. What STD the patient has, its implications and treatment, and the importance of complying with treatment.
2. The patient's risk level.
3. The need to change sexual behaviour.
4. Any barriers the patient may have to changing risky behaviour.
5. What changes the patient can and will make in their sexual behaviour.
6. The need to treat sexual partners.

This list also offers a sensible order in which to cover the points. We need to explore each one in more detail.

1. Explaining the STD and its treatment

The first step is to:

- explain what STD the patient has, and what treatment is necessary - the name of the drug and how much to take, for how long. Write down these details for the patient - or use recognizable symbols if the patient cannot read;
- find out what the patient understands about the STD and its treatment, and what questions and concerns he or she may have;
- advise about any common side-effects of the treatment;
- encourage the patient to comply with treatment.

In Workbook 4 we stressed the importance of using language that the patient can understand. Only use medical terms if you are sure that the patient knows them, otherwise remember to use words that are meaningful to him or her.

ACTIVITY

What words are commonly used to describe these syndromes in your region, and what do people believe causes them?

Syndrome	*Regional name or description*	*Cause*
Vaginal discharge		
Urethral discharge		

Genital ulcers

Scrotal swelling

---

lower abdominal pain

Inguinal bubo

Neonatal conjunctivitis

As with all treatments, it is essential that the patient completes the recommended treatment, even if their symptoms disappear or they feel better. Remind them that the symptoms will recur if they do not take all the medication.

2. The patient's risk level

Once you are sure the patient understands what STD they have, and what treatment to follow, he or she must next appreciate what risk there is of becoming re-infected. For you, there are two stages to this issue: first, assessing the patient's risk level, and secondly explaining it to the patient.

High-risk behaviour is behaviour that exposes the patient to infected blood, semen, vaginal fluid or genital lesions.

Assessing the patient's risk level

If as in most cases, you have already taken the patient's history, you may have enough information to assess the risk of re-infection. The next page contains a list of possible issues that may help you confirm the risks.

ACTIVITY

Please read through the issues on the next page and mark any that you think may not be relevant when assessing a patient's risk of STD infection. Use the space below to make notes, and discuss your reasons with a colleague.

Assessing the patient's risk of further STD

Personal sexual behaviour:

1. Number of sexual partners in the past year.
2. Sex with a new or different partner in the post three months.
3. Any other STD in the post year.
4. Has the patient ever exchanged sex for money, goods or drugs (include both giving and receiving)?
5. Use of herbs as a drying agent, or similar sexual practices.

Partner(s) sexual behaviour:

Does the patient's partners):

- have sex with other partners?
- also have an STD?
- have HIV-infection?
- inject drugs?
- If male have sex with other men?

Personal Drug use:

The key issue is whether the patient is mixing drugs with sex - which may increase the risk of spreading STD or being re-infected. Sharing needles or 'works' also carries a high risk of transmitting or being infected with HIV, so:

1. Use of alcohol or other drugs (if so, what?), before or during sex?
2. Exchange of sex for drugs (or drugs for sex)?

Other personal risk factors:

1. HIV infection?
2. Use of skin-piercing instruments such as:
   - needles (injections, tattoos);

- scarification or body-piercing tools;
- circumcision Knives;

3. Has the patient ever had a blood transfusion? When?
4. For young children, risk of perinatul transmission of STD/HIV means that service providers must question the parents about their possible infections, for example, gonorrhoea, syphilis, chlamydia, HIV.

Patient's protective behaviour:

1. What does the patient do to protect him/herself from STD/HIV?
2. Use of condoms? When and how? How often? With whom?
3. What kinds of low-risk or safe sexual activities does the patient practise? How often? With whom? Why?

IMPORTANT POINTS

Many of these questions were included in Section 3 of Workbook 3: don't ask questions to which you already have the answers. Also, as you learn about a patient's sexual experience, you may find that some questions are not relevant

Helping the patient identify his/her risk factors

Once you have a clear idea of the patient's risk level, the next step is to help the patient understand what risks they are taking in their present sexual behoviour, and which behaviours are safer.

Help the patient identify what risks he or she has been taking in the past, then work together to explore options for safer sex. Safer options might include:

1. Limiting sexual partners to one faithful partner.
2. Using condoms consistently and correctly.
3. Reporting high-risk penetrative (sex such as unprotected vaginal or anal intercourse) with low-risk non-penetrative sex (such as mutual masturbation)

At any time when discussing sexual behaviour with a patient, check for misconceptions. Few patients have a *complete* or *accurate* picture of either the causes of STD or how to avoid infection. Accurate information is often mixed with local beliefs. Clearly, patients with inaccurate beliefs about the causes of STD may have a false sense of security - and run an even greater risk of re-infection with STD. Some common beliefs about STD/HIV include:

* the idea that certain people, such as married women, young girls or boys or 'clean' partners, are usually free from infection;
* taking anti-malorials before or after sex offers protection;

"urinating, washing or douching after sex protects against STD;

* the patient's belief that he/she does not belong to a high-risk group (such as commercial sex workers or homosexual males) so he/she is safe.

QUESTION

3. *Note* down any common beliefs *about* protection against STD *in your region.*

Making sure that the patient understands that he or she became infected by unprotected sexual intercourse with an infected partner, and that there are no other causes.

3. The need to change sexual behaviour

The patient now knows how he or she was infected by an STD and is also aware of the risk of re-infection. The third, fourth and fifth steps are about helping the patient to change his or her sexual behaviour-perhaps the service provider's most challenging task. Dividing one issue into three enables you to take a decision-making approach with the patient.

This step means helping the patent decide to change his or her sexual behaviour in order to avoid further infection. It is a good idea to give the patient the opportunity to identify what changes might be possible in his or her own life.

Remember the three main safe behaviours we discussed in step 2. Any one of these behaviours is appropriate, and more than one if the patient has sex with a variety of different partners.

4. Barriers to changing behoviour

All health providers are aware of the difficulty of changing behaviour. Life would be easy if people responded to health messages by doing as they were advised, but many don't. Why? Because awareness of the health message is not enough. To make real changes, we need first to overcome 'barriers' in our life and experience.

1. Gender raises real borders. These arise, essentially, from the power imbalance between men and women and from the different expectations and values relating to male and female sexuality. Women often have very little control over when, with

whom, and under what circumstances they have sex. They are therefore not in a position to protect themselves, even if they so wish or have the means (e.g. a condom).

2 Cultural practices may help or hinder the patient's ability to change. Consider the possible barriers relating to age differences at marriage, wife inheritance, puberty rites, sexuality, child-rearing and so on, as well as the values of family and community.

3. Religion may under some circumstances contribute to adoption of safer sexual behaviour. However, it poses major barriers to change in that it discourages open discussion about sexuality and some protective measures.

4. Poverty, social disruption and civil unrest force women and girls in particular, but, sometimes, boys into exchanging sex for material favours or even for survival. In less extreme situations, lock of access to education and employment may force women to exchange sex with a number of partners in order to pay for food, shelter and clothing for themselves and their children.

Please consider these three questions, perhaps with colleagues.

a) How might factors like the ones we have listed create barriers to change in your region?

---

b) What other barriers might apply? For instance, what social norms can you think of that interfere with changing sexual behaviour?

---

c) To what extent do these barriers vary between men and women, or between people of different ages?

---

5. Changes the patient will make in their sexual behaviour

Having asked the patient to identify ways they might change, and explored any barriers to doing so, you can now help the patient to decide which change would be easiest and/or most effective in their own life - and how to put it into practice.

The change most likely to succeed is the one that fits most easily with the patient's present lifestyle, once you have helped the patient to overcome any relevant barriers.

A useful approach might be to help the patient to analyse the costs and benefits of changing their behaviour. Typically, existing behaviour has the benefit of no change and the *cost* of further STD infection. In contrast, the change in sexual behoviour has the benefit of protection against STD but a number of possible costs, from the price of condoms to the patient's need to ask a partner to use condoms.

It is not quite enough simply to have the patient agree the chosen safe behaviour Ask him or her how they will put it into practice, when they will do so, and what they will do if, for any reason, they do practise risky sex. These are difficult issues, but we will explore some useful skills for you in the next section of this workbook.

6. The need to treat sexual partners

This is the theme of Workbook 6, so we need not discuss it in any detail here. Remember: always tell your patient how important it is to have all their known partners treated, and that they risk re-infection otherwise unless they use condom consistently. Reassure the patient that you will maintain their confidentiality, and discuss how they can persuade the partner or partners to attend for treatment.

That almost brings us to the end of this first section. Please try the questions on the next page to help you check what you have learned and apply some of the ideas.

4. *Imagine you have taken the history and assessed the risks for each of the four STD patients that follow. On the basis of the information you have been given, make notes in answer to these two questions:*

- *what risk behaviours should the patient aim to avoid in the future?*
- *what barriers to change might arise from the patient's circumstances?*

a) *Nina is a 19-year-old commercial sex worker who lives in a slum area of town. She has one small child who is often sick. Nina is also using her earnings to help support her family who live in a remote village. Her family disapprove of her job but eagerly accept the money that she sends home. She is afraid of AIDS but finds that many of her clients refuse to use condoms. You have diagnosed a genital ulcer.*

b) *John a 24-year-old single man with a good job and his own home. He doesn't want to settle down for a long time, describing himself as 'a good time guy'. He has three sexual partners and sometimes has casual sex too. However, he says he chooses women who are 'clean' or 'married', so he can't understand why he now has a urethral discharge. During the interview he admits that he often gets drunk or injects drugs with one of his partners before sex.*

c) ***Amina** is 35, married with three teenage children. She relies on her husband's income from factory work to support the family. During the interview, she said that she has sex only with her husband. She responded to your questions by saying that her husband often worked late at the factory, and that he went for a drink with friends occasionally: she could smell the alcohol on his breath. However she feels quite secure in his faithfulness to her. She came to the centre with no idea of the cause of her abdominal pain - you have diagnosed pelvic inflammatory disease.*

---

d) ***Tony** is a 47-year-old married man, living in a rural area. His eldest brother died recently and everyone in the family suspects that he died of AIDS. His culture and religion dictate that Tony will inherit his brother's 36-year-old wife, taking her as his second wife. He has heard a lot about AIDS on the radio, and so is fearful that he and his first wife might be exposed to AIDS or STD. Presenting initially with bad head pains, Tony has really come to ask your help in resolving this problem.*

Summary

In this first part of Section, B, we have explored the six issues that you need to explore with an STD patient:

1. What STD the patient has, its implications and treatment, and the importance of complying with treatment.
2. The patient's risk level, which you may need to learn about by careful, sympathetic questioning, and which you should then discuss with the patient.
3. The patient's need to change their sexual behoviour, and what safe sex behaviours might be appropriate to their lifestyle.
4. Any barriers the patient may have to changing behaviour: if you cannot help the patient overcome these barriers, they are unlikely to change their sexual behaviour.
5. What changes the patient can and will make in their sexual behaviour: those to which you can help the patient feel committed.
6. The need to treat sexual partners, and how to achieve this objective while ensuring the patient's confidence.

What we have left out so far is the reaction of individual patients to these messages: their feelings and real difficulties. But, as you know from Module 3, it is essential always to work with the patient's feelings, to provide reassurance and respect.

Please note down any questions or concerns that you have now that you have completed Section 1, then discuss them with your colleagues or trainer. Please also discuss the activity questions with colleagues if you have not already done so.

C. EDUCATE-HOW?

In Section 1, you worked through the many complex issues that the patient with STD needs to confront. In this section we answer the question: how do you educate and support the patient?

Your learning objectives

By the end of this section, you will be able to:

- define education in the context of STD case management;
- appreciate why education is so important for patients with STD;
- identify a range of useful skills that will enable you to educate and support the patient effectively.

In Section 1, you identified all the issues that patients need to learn about. You learned that they also need to make three essential decisions: to comply with treatment, to change sexual behaviour, and to have sexual partners treated.

Is it enough to simply *inform* a patient about all these issues and urge him or he to comply with your suggestions? No! As many as 70% of all patients may fail to comply with treatment advice, even when the advice is given clearly and accurately.

So information and advice is not enough. We need to educate each patient. In fact, education is crucial to the success of syndromic management of STD.

Education is part of a process of enabling someone to change, to make choices and decisions. And, in order to change, the patient must want to change.

How do we achieve that desire to change?

In a number of ways.

First, it is important to use the communication skills you developed with Workbook 3: open questions, facilitation, summarising and checking, reassurance, direction, empathy and partnership. These are essential for the many times that you will ask questions or help the patient deal with emotions.

As you move into education and the need to motivate the patient to changes, these are the additional skills you will need:

- explanation and instruction
- modelling
- reinforcing strengths you see in the patient
- helping the patient explore choices
- rehearsing what the patient will do or say
- confirming the patient's decisions

We will explore each of these skills in turn, illustrating each one with examples from two of the case studies at the end of Section: John and Amina.

Amina's interview in particular illustrates the powerful feelings of shock and hurt that news of an STD can bring. For some patients this comes from a sense of personal shame; for others it may be caused by the collapse of security or trust in a long-term relationship. Whatever the source of these feelings, the service provider must be able to manage them in order to help the patient change his or her sexual behaviour or persuade his/her partner to do so.

> *This workbook cannot help you become a fully trained counselor. If you have already had any training in educating or counselling patients, you should already have the above skills and more. Use this section to refresh your understanding of the skills, and please be willing to help any colleagues practise them.*

Explanation and instruction

These are skills that many service providers use most of the time.

Instruction	Telling patients what to do or how to do something, such as use a condom or take medication: "Remember to complete the whole course of tablets, right to the last one..."
Explanation	Telling patients how or why something should be done: "You have pain low in your tummy because of an infection passed to you during sexual intercourse ..."

Even here it may be possible to develop your skills a little more. For example:

- are you communicating clearly and simply?
- do you adapt your pace and language to the needs of the patient?

How can you find out if you are communicating effectively? The best way is to provide the patient with time to ask questions. If the patient seems anxious or confused, stop and check: "Is what I'm saying making sense to you?". And ask the patient to summarise what you've said: "I've covered a lot of information and I want to be sure I've done so clearly. Please tell me what you need to do in your own words".

The news that an infection is sexually transmitted might shock some patients. How could you 'break the news' to such a person tactfully yet clearly?

Please discuss this question with your colleagues.

In the first section we stressed the importance of asking the patient for their opinions. For example, in explaining risk behaviour, we suggested that it would be useful to ask the patient what behaviour they thought risked STD infection. So as often as you con, ask the patient what they already know before explaining something in detail. Here's an example from Amina's interview.

Service provider	*Please don't worry Amina, I'm going to help you all I can. Your illness is caused by an infection. Do you know how you got the infection?*
Amina	*Well, I 'm not sure but . . . um . . .*
Service provider	Yes?
Amina	*Well, perhaps it's something I ate?*
Service provider	*I'm afraid not. This is going to be difficult news for you. ... You have pelvic inflammatory disease. It's a sexually transmitted disease. Do you know what that means?*
Amina	*Well, that comes from touching dirty people ... but it can't be that.*

Service provider *You 're right, it's not that.... but perhaps you'll think this is worse. Illnesses like this one are only caused by having unprotected sex with someone else who has the same illness. Unprotected sex means sex without a condom.*

Amina *But I only make love with my husband. He's not ill ...*

Service provider *He doesn't necessarily have to feel ill, Amina. People often don't. But if you've been faithful to him, then he must have passed the infection to you. And he must have got the infection ...*

Amina *From sex with someone else? No ... No.*

Service provider *You're very upset at this news, I can see. You need time to think about it.*

Notice how carefully the service provider is introducing this news to Amina. She is breaking her explanation into very small steps in order to work with Amina's feelings.

We can summarise a useful approach to explanation as:

1. Ask for the patient's ideas (e.g. diagnosis).
2. Discuss the patient's ideas.
3. Explain the subject.
4. Check the patient's understanding and feelings.

You might like to go back to the interview extract on page 18 and underline phrases you think useful. Alternatively, practise identifying where the service provider is explaining something, and where he/she is using other communication skills.

Modelling

This skill enables you to present examples of how the recommended behaviour or treatment has been successful in other cases. Here is part of John's interview:

John *Can't I ever have some fun without risking this again?*

Service provider *Of course you can have fun. It just needs to take a new form. It's hard to change, so let's talk about how you can be safer.*

John Are you saying there's something wrong with having a drink first and stuff?

Service provider	Only because drinking tends to make people forgetful. It's hard enough to get used to a condom, but if you're drinking it's even harder to remember to use one. I want you to know that I've noticed more guys are being careful - and they still have their 'fun ' even while being safe. I've seen lots of guys lately who have decided to drink less and use a condom.

Notice that modelling also helps to stress your positive experience: "From my work I know ..." or "I've noticed that ..." for example.

Why is this positive modelling so important? We know that the alternative is to tell any STD patient "If you don't do this you may get AIDS and die!". While such words of doom may contain some truth, we also know that they aren't very successful in persuading people to change their behaviour. Focusing on *positive* outcomes of change is a much more successful approach.

Reinforcing strengths

This means pointing out a strength or positive attribute that you see in the patient - something that will help him or her recover or prevent the recurrence of STD.

John	*OK, likeI know it's important but ... I don't think I could get used to it at all ...*
Service provider	*It's hard but I noticed you walked 10 kilometers to get here for treatment of your infection. Your determination and concern will help you to be safe.*

Reinforcing strengths could be really useful in helping Amina to manage her feelings so that the service provider can direct her back to treatment:

Amina	*I feel ... as if my whole life has been broken. I can't cope with all this ...what am I going to do?*
Service provider	*I appreciate your feelings Amina. Your sense of trust has been broken. You clearly care for your husband and family very much, and those feelings will help you to get through the next few days ... but first, let's talk about how we can get you better!*
Amina	*Yes, yes you're right of course. I've got to think about this for a while: are you going to give me some tablets?*

Exploring choices

The provider points out alternative choices or steps that the patient can take towards achieving the goal of curing the current STD or preventing another one. He or she then helps the patient to decide which is best.

John	*So it's condoms or* one partner or *sex without intercourse. . .*
Service provider	*That's right. You can either settle down with one partner or, if you 're not ready for that, protect yourself with condoms or non-penetrative sex. Which will be easiest for you right now?*
John Condoms	*I suppose. I'm not going to settle down yet!*

Offering a choice also empowers the patient, who feels more in control of the decision that he/she will make. The patient may have a sense of 'ownership' of the decision:

Service provider	*For today Amina, I'd like you to make a choice. Would you prefer to avoid sex until you have* finished the *treatment, or to* ask *your husband to use condoms?*
Amina	*That's easy: no sex for a while. That won't be a problem because he knows I'm not feeling well. It'll give me time to think about things a bit.*
Service provider	*Yes, it will: that's a good idea.*

Rehearsing decisions

When you feel sure that the patient has reached a decision on the appropriate safe behaviourts), it is important to ask him or her to work through the steps that will put the decision into practice. Here are two examples:

Service provider	*Very good John. How are you going to explain this to your girlfriends?*
John	*Well, I could start* by *saying there* are *lots of* bad *diseases around, and that we must be careful to avoid them.*
Service provider	*That sounds great. Go on.*
Service provider	*So, you're planning to avoid sex until you've finished*

	the tablets. Your husband needs to be treated as well ... how will you approach him about it?
Amina	*I need to talk to him about a few things. I mean, is it something serious or is he just playing around? Or perhaps I'll just ask him to come and see you ...so you can treat him ...*

Rehearsal is also useful when you want to check that the patient has understood your instructions on treatment.

Confirming decisions

This is a very useful way of concluding the interview. You have helped the patient understand a number of issues and to prepare for what they will do after leaving the health centre. Asking the patient to confirm a decision helps him or her to feel motivated on leaving the centre. Having reinforced their decision to you, they are much more likely to practise safer sex than before:

Service provider	*Well, John, I think that's about everything. Just tell me once more what you intend to do with these tablets.*
John	*I'm going to take all of them just as I've got on this piece of paper - I'll keep the paper in this pocket - and I'm not going with my girlfriends until I've finished them...but I'll buy some condoms just in case.*
Service provider	*You're being very brave, Amina, and that's important. Go over your plans with me once again.*
Amina	*Get better, take all the tablets, find time to talk to my* husband about a few things. And he needs treatment too. . .
Service provider	*Yes, well done. And you will come and see me again if you need to?*
Amina	*Yes. I will.*

Summary

The goal of educating STD patients is to enable them to make informed decisions to change their sexual behaviour. Both the issues in Section -C and the skills in Section are designed to help you move the patient towards decisions.

Education issues

1. The STD, its implications and treatment, and the importance of *complying* with treatment.
2. The patient's risk level.
3. The need to change sexual behaviour.
4. Barriers the patient may have to changing behaviour.
5. What changes the patient can and will make in their sexual behaviour.
6. The need to treat sexual partners.

Education and motivation skills

Explanation and instruction.
Modelling .
Reinforcing strengths.
Exploring choices.
Rehearsing decisions.
Confirming decisions.

Notice that, while you need to cover the issues roughly in the order above, you can draw on any of the skills as you need them.

Also, as you saw in Amina's interview, dealing with the patient's feelings is an essential part of this process, so you will often need to draw on your communication skills.

As with history-taking, it is important to practise all these skills. Please turn now to the Action Plan which begins on the next page.

D. ACTION PLAN 1

Please find time soon to practise the skills you have studied so far.

If you are studying with a group of people as part of a course, your trainer will guide the role ploy and explain what you have to do.

If you are studying on your own, follow the guidance below very carefully and, if possible, ask two other service providers to work on the role plays with you. They should either be studying the programme or be already trained in syndromic case management of STD.

The aim of this role play is to practise the necessary skills and issues for educating and counselling patients up to the point when the patient has understood step 3: the *need* to *change sexual behaviour, including what constitutes risky and safe sexual behaviour.* This will enable you to:

- apply effective communication skills when educating patients about STD;
- clarify areas on which you want to work further in order to refine your skills.

To practise without a trainer, three people need to take part. In each role play, one person should be the patient, one the service provider, and the third person should observe the role-play and provide constructive feedback to help the 'service provider' develop his or her skills. Here is what to do.

1. Please read the four case studies in order to get a general picture of each patient described. There is no need to take notes or develop any of the case studies. Remember that the service provider has already taken the patient's history and diagnosed the STD.
2. Decide who will first be the patient, the service provider and the observer.
3. The patient should select one of the case studies. Base your selection on the study that represents a patient similar to one you commonly see in your clinical setting or that presents issues you want to learn to deal with more effectively. Tell the others which case study you have selected.
4. Prepare for the role play by studying the guidance–for the patient, for the service provider and for the observer.
5. When the role play is completed and each of you is satisfied that you have given or received sufficient feedback, swap roles and repeat steps 2 - 4 above, so that each learner has the opportunity to practise education skills.

Preparing to be the patient

Please reread your selected case study very carefully, because your aim is to respond as realistically and honestly as you can to whatever the service provider says and does. Do not try to make it either easy or difficult for him or her.

1. Based on the limited information you have about the patient, decide in advance what factual information you may need to answer the provider's questions. Common questions might be about how many partners you have, whether you use condoms regularly and what you know about the transmission of STD.
2. Note your feelings as this patient. For example, how do you feel while waiting for your diagnosis? What questions, if any, do you have for the service provider? What is worrying you?
3. During the role ploy, identify as much as you can with how this patient would behave. Use empathy to experience what the patient might feel in this situation.

4. After the role play, explain how you experienced the interview. It is important to provide feedback, both on what worked well and what didn't. For example, you might tell the service provider you felt reassured by the way they spoke to you softly so that others would not hear, and that you only wish they had given you more time to talk about your feelings about having the STD ... that you felt a little rushed at times.

   Very specific feedback is also helpful for the provider, such as "I didn't understand when it was time to put on the condom... right away or just before the man wants to have intercourse, or what?".
5. As the service provider and observer review the exercise, feel free to add any useful insights you have into the service provider's behaviour. At this point, make sure that your suggestions are positive ones that will help the service provider to usefully develop his or her skills.

Case study 1: Nina

Nina is a 1 9-year-old commercial sex worker who lives in a slum area of town. She has one small child who is often sick. Nina has no partner. She is also using her earnings to help support her family who live in a remote village. Her family disapprove of her job but eagerly accept the money that she sends home. She is afraid of AIDS but finds that many of her clients refuse to use condoms; she also has a limited knowledge about STD. The service provider has diagnosed a genital ulcer; Nina is afraid it might be an STD.

Case study 2: John

John is a 24-year-old single man with a good job and his own home. He does not want to settle down for a long time, describing himself as 'a good time guy'. He has three sexual partners and sometimes has casual sex too. However, he says he chooses women who are 'clean' or 'married', so he can't understand why he now has a urethral discharge. During the interview he admits that he often gets drunk or injects drugs with one of his partners before sex. The service provider has confirmed the urethral discharge.

____

____

____

____

____

____

Case study 3: Amina

Amina is 35, married with three teenage children. She relies on her husbands income from factory work to support the family. During the interview, she said that she has sex only with her husband. She has already explained that her husband often works late at the factory, and that he goes for a drink with friends occasionally: she can sometimes smell the alcohol on his breath. However she feels quite secure in his faithfulness to her. She came to the centre with no idea of the cause of her abdominal pain - the service provider has diagnosed pelvic inflammatory disease.

____

____

____

____

____

____

____

Case study 4: Ahmed

Ahmed is 35, married with four children and living in a rural area. He attended an urban clinic with a swelling in his groin which the service provider diagnosed as an inguinal bubo. In answering the service provider's questions, he admitted reluctantly that he has sex with a number of other partners, many of them causal, in the course of his search for work. He regularly travels to the city, working away from home for three months at a time. He says that his wife is currently six months pregnant: he has not been home for two months though he regularly sends home money. He is currently living with a casual partner in the city.

____

____

____

____

____

____

The service provider's role

Your overall aim is to obtain clear feedback on your present skills and areas that you might usefully rehearse or refine.

During the role play, your aim is to obtain the patient's compliance on treatments and their understanding of safe sex that will prevent future infections. In other words, go no further through the issues than step 3: the need to change sexual behaviour. (The second role play at the back of the workbook will complete the education process.)

Remember to use your skills in education and motivation to help the patient make choices and confirm any decisions.

1. Review the skills and themes that the observer will be looking for in your interview.
2. Reread the patient's selected case study to familiarise yourself with what you have already learned while taking their history. If you wish, make notes on key questions you want to ask.
3. Conduct the interview, starting with your discussion about what STD the patient has, and stopping when you feel sure that the patient understands high-risk and safe sexual behaviour - or after the agreed time if that comes first.
4. After the role play, allow the patient to give you feedback on

how he/she felt during the interview. Next, give your own views and feelings about how the education process went. Finally, the observer will provide feedback based on the checklists he or she is using. Feel free to ask either the patient or observer to clarify what they have said: you want to finish the role play with helpful objectives and, hopefully, confirmation of your perceived strengths!

The observer's role

Your aim is, after the role play, to provide the service provider with clear, objective feedback on what they achieved during this education part of the interview.

1. Read through the checklist below to familiarise yourself with the skills and issues that the service provider should use.
2. Time the interview, stopping it after an agreed time, such as 5 minutes.
3. As you observe, make quick notes on the skills you see the service provider use, and how effectively you think he/she uses them. If possible, note examples of what he/she said or did so that your feedback will be as practical as possible.
4. Ask the patient, and then the service provider to review the interview. Start your feedback by responding briefly to the service provider's self-criticism, and then give your own feedback, skill by skill or however else you think appropriate. Be willing to give negative criticism if necessary, but offer it in a constructive way: "When the patient said ... you said ... Perhaps it would have helped if ..." and so on. Always stress the provider's positive achievements and be as practical as you can. For example, suggest alternative ways the provider could have introduced specific issues, or ask him/her to identify when one skill might have been more appropriate than the one used.
5. Finally, lead a discussion about what the three of you have learned from the role play. There might be a number of valid issues that this workbook has not included.

Observation checklist

To what extent does the service provider:

a) Cover these education issues?

---

1. The STD, its implications and treatment, and the importance of *complying* with treatment

2. The patient's risk level

3. The need to change sexual behaviour and what constitutes safe sex

b) Use these education and motivation skills?
1. Explanation and instruction
2. Modelling
3. Reinforcing strengths
4. Exploring choices
5. Rehearsing decisions
6. Confirming decisions

c) Apply these communication skills?
1. Facilitation
2. Summarising and checking
3. Reassurance
4. Direction
5. Empathy
6. Partnership

E. USING CONDOMS TO STAY CURED

This section will enable you to:
- list the benefits of using a condom;
- demonstrate how to use a condom;
- explain how to keep and dispose of condoms.

As you know, condoms help people to have safer sex by preventing contact between vaginal fluids and semen or blood. Using condoms is especially important if your patient has sex with more than one partner or with one partner who has other sexual partners. However it is not enough to know that condoms are important. Patients must also know how to use them properly.

Many people resist the idea of using condoms, not only because of the embarrassment or cost of buying them. For instance, they think that condoms spoil sex or that they are too big or too small. And there are often myths about them - such as rumours that condoms are not effective or that the condom itself is infected with STD! They may also associate them with illicit sex - rather than for use with a regular partner.

Are there any 'myths' about condoms in your region, and if so, what are they? Who holds these beliefs?

It is important to be aware of negative ideas about condoms because, clearly, they would form a barrier to the patient's willingness to comply with safe sexual behaviour. You also need to explain that condoms work well if used properly and consistently. Describe the benefits of using condoms most relevant to the individual patient.

5. *What do you think are the advantages of using condoms? Note down as many ideas as you can below:*

Condoms are an important option for anyone who has sex with more than one partner or whose partner may be doing so. So how can you persuade someone to seriously consider them? Of course, the first step is to convince yourself of the benefits !

As well as stressing their benefits, use all the skills we have discussed in Section as well as your general communication skills. In other words, ask the patient what they think of condoms, discuss their response and any barriers towards using them, and suggest appropriate benefits. If the patient continues to resist their use, repeat the other forms of safe sex and ask if one of them would be preferable:

John	*You said condoms is one way of keeping safe, but I wouldn 't use them.*

Service provider *Why not?*
John *Well, they're a nuisance. I mean they get in the way, if you know what I mean.*
Service provider *So you have tried to use them before?*
John *Well, no. But I've been told that.*
Service provider Well, they needn't get in the way. I can show you how to use them. I know a lot of men who have fun with them because they ask their partners to put it on for them.
John *Yes, but what if it comes off?*
Service provider *It can 't come off if you use it properly, I promise you. Any other reasons for not liking them?*
John *No, that's the main thing.*
Service provider *Some men say that condoms can actually make intercourse last longer. What do you think of that?*
John *{Laughs embarrassedly) Sounds OK.*
Service provider *Would you be willing* to try *using* them?
John *OK, I could* give them a try.
Service provider *Good - but remember, if you don 't use condoms, you must stick with one partner or practise non-penetrative sex. Let me show you how to use a condom.*

Demonstrating the use of condoms

Please look at Figure 1 on the next page, which illustrates some of the main steps in correct use of a condom.

It is important to first demonstrate its use and then ask the patient to practise the same method, helping him or her to get it right. This means that you will need a supply of condoms and a penis model or something to represent one, such as a banana or broom handle.

In your demonstration:

- stress the importance of carrying condoms all the time - the patient should never be without one;
- show the expiry or manufacture date and explain that the condom should not be out-of-date, smelly, sticky or hard to unroll;
- explain how to open the package carefully, using the test-point;
- show the correct side of the condom to insert over the penis, explaining that it won't roll down if placed the other way;
- show how to hold the tip of the condom to press out air, before rolling it all the way down the erect penis;
- emphasize that the condom must be rolled right down to its base;

How to use Condom

1. Check the expiry date and the manufacture date.

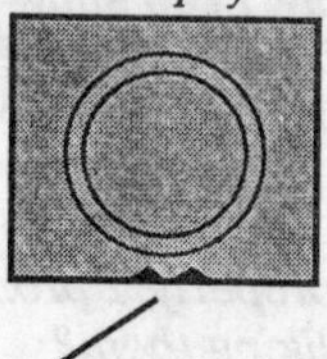

2. Tear the wrapper carefully.

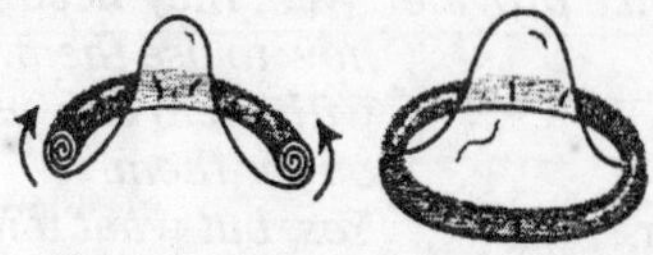

3. Hold the condom this way up so that it will unravel easily.

4. Holding the top of the condom, press out the air from the tip and roll the condom on. Use both hands.

5. Roll the condom right to the base of the penis, leaving space at the tip of the condom for semen.

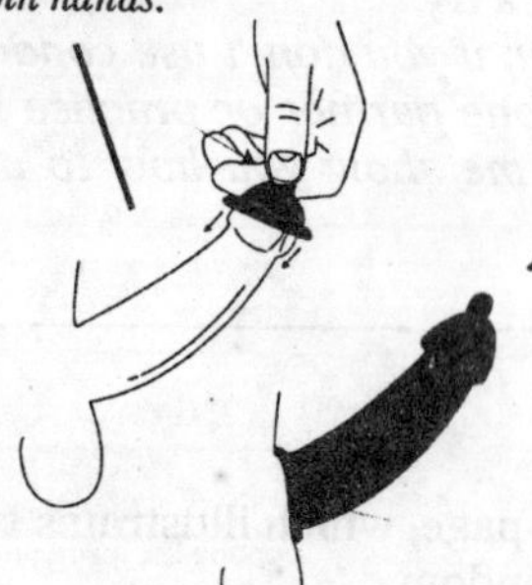

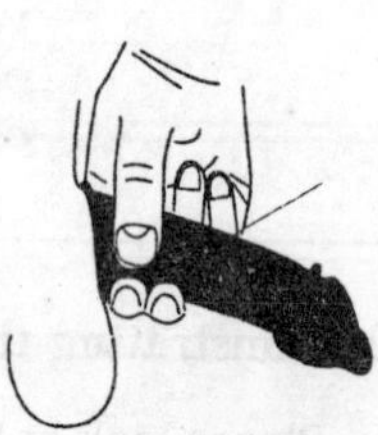

6. After ejaculation, when you sturt losing erection, hold the condom at the bose and slide it corefully off.

- explain that the condom should be removed *just as the penis begins to lose its erection,* and that the patient should hold it carefully at the base and slide it off slowly;
- explain that, to dispose of it safely, the patient should tie the top and dispose of it safely.

There are two other tips you might want to give the patient:

- do not use oil or oil-based lubricants such as petroleum jelly, which damage latex condoms (water-based lubricants such as glycerin and K-Y Jelly are safe, as are most spermicidal foams);
- do not reuse condoms.

6. *A young man with an STD tells you impatiently: "I already; know how to use condoms! What's the point of demonstrating it to me?" What might you say to him?*

7. *There are many myths about condom use. Which of the following statements are true or false? Circle the responses you think are correct.*

a) *Condoms can get lost inside the woman.*

TRUE *FALSE*

b} *Condoms don't protect against STD including HIV.*

TRUE *FALSE*

c) *Condoms can be kept in a pocket or wallet indefinitely.*

TRUE *FALSE*

d) *It is OK to use glycerin or water-based lubricants with condoms.*

TRUE FALSE

e) *Pull the condom tight over the head of the penis to ensure a snug fit.*

TRUE *FALSE*

f) *Squeeze the air out of the tip of the condom as you put it on.*

TRUE *FALSE*

g) *Condoms should be stored in a cool, dark, dry place.*

TRUE FALSE

Summary

In this *section we have explored:*

- the benefits of using condoms, and some of the negatively ideas about them that you might have to confront;
- how to demonstrate their use and what advice to give the patient.

Remember: you need also to use *all the* communication and education skills you have learned so for when discussing *and* demonstrating condoms.

Ideally, health centres could provide patients with free condoms. If this is not possible, make sure you know the answers to questions like these, so that you can advise your patients accordingly:

Where can the patient buy condoms?
How much do they cost?
Are they of good quality?
Are different sizes available?

F. REVIEW

Now that you have completed Workbook 5, you should be able to:

- explain why education and emotional support are vital in the management of STD;
- identify six main issues on which you need to educate and motivate patients;
- identify six skills that will help you to educate and motivate patients;
- demonstrate the use of condoms and explain their benefits.

The next step is very important because you need to practise what you have learned. Action Plan 2 will help you to do this.

G. ACTION PLAN 2

The aim of this Action Plan is to practise educating patients on all the remaining issues, including the use of condoms. The only issue to leave out is the sixth one treating the patient's sexual partners.

If you are studying with a group of learners and a trainer, then your trainer will guide you on this role play.

If you are studying on your own, please arrange to work with two other service providers just as you did before - preferably they should be the same people as for Action Plan 1.

Take up the some case studies as before, at the point where the role ploys finished last time. This should be at the point where the patient has understood what is meant by safe sexual behaviour. The service provider's remaining tasks are these:

4. To identify any barriers the patient may have to changing current behavior
5. To help the patient identify appropriate changes and decide which one(s) they will adopt as new safe behaviour.

This should include using condoms, in which the service provider should educate the patient on relevant personal benefits as well as demonstrating how to use them.

Please arrange your role ploys exactly as you did for Action Plan 1, except that, this time the 'service provider' can concentrate on developing particular skills identified during his/her role play and feedback. The observer should look for the same educational and communication skills, and concentrate on the issues above.

H. OTHER OPPORTUNITIES FOR PATIENT EDUCATION: ASSIGNMENT

The health centre could offer many opportunities to reinforce and supplement the service provider's efforts at patient education. These opportunities could be provided by people in different areas of the centre as well as by a range of media.

You might like to consider other opportunities for patient education within your health centre. Here are some suggestions:

Who? All staff who meet patients can assist with patient education. For example, staff at reception might contribute by demonstrating respect, empathy and reassurance - which maintains patients' dignity and reduces any fear or shame they might be feeling.

Where? Patient education can take place at each step that patients go through during a visit to the health centre, from the registration desk to the waiting room, the examination or interview room and the dispensary.

How? A health centre can draw on a wide range of media for its education process, limited only by the resources available. To name a few:

- posters
- brochures, leaflets to be read on-site or taken away as handouts
- audio tapes playing
- video tapes playing
- small group discussions and more formal health talks
- condom demonstrations
- drama presentations by local theatre groups or health educators

Walk round your health centre as if you were a patient coming in for treatment.

What opportunities for patient education does the centre use?

What opportunities could the centre usefully adopt for patient education?

- How would your suggestion contribute to effective patient education at the centre?
- Who could be responsible for developing this suggestion?
- What resources would be needed?

Please discuss your suggestions with your trainer or supervisor.

I. ANSWERS

1 a) The two types of question we were thinking of are open and closed questions. Well done if you remembered the advantages of open questions during most of the interview. They enable the patient to express concerns in their own language, and often mean for fewer questions need to be asked. Closed questions are useful to obtain specific extra details later in the interview.

b) These are the six verbal skills we suggested:
- facilitation;
- summarising and checking;
- reassurance;
- direction;
- empathy;
- partnership.

Don't worry if you only remembered one or two of these skills. The important thing is that you use them when interviewing patients!

2. In fact, at this stage in the interview there are six issues to discuss with the patient:
   1. What STD the patient has, its implications and treatment, and the importance of *complying* with treatment.
   2. The patient's risk level.
   3. The need to change sexual behaviour.
   4. Any barriers the patient may have to changing risky behaviour.
   5. What changes the patient can and will make in their sexual behaviour.
   6 The need to treat sexual partners.

In addition, with female patients who are pregnant, you may need to discuss the need to protect the baby.

3. Please discuss this question with your colleagues because it is important to be aware of the predominant local beliefs about STD. These are some of the more frequently found beliefs that are important to understand and address:
   - one STD can turn into another one;
   - you can only get one STD at a time;

- all STDs, including HIV, are detected using one diagnostic test;
- health care personnel can tell if a patient has STD without testing,
- people with STDs always have symptoms;
- you can't have STD and HIV at the some time;
- you can tell who has an STD/HIV by how he or she looks or feels;
- you can tell who has an STD/HIV by their actions, occupation, social close or number of sex partners.

4. Don't worry if you found this exercise difficult or if your answers differ slightly from ours, below. You may well have considered issues equally relevant to ours: if at all unsure, talk to an experienced colleague.

    a) The risk behaviour of which we are aware is Nina's occupation, which involves sleeping with a number of casual partners. We do not know whether she mixes sex with alcohol or drug consumption: the service provider would need to check this out with her.

    Nina's barriers to change? Two major ones: Her reliance on sex as her only source of income to support her child and family, and her inability to persuade clients to use condoms. Presumably she feels that she cannot afford to lose clients by insisting on this.

    b) John's risk behaviour includes alcohol and drug use as well as unprotected sex with a number of partners, including casual partners of whose sexual practices he knows nothing. He also has an incorrect idea about safe sexual behaviour which gives him a false sense of security.

    Barriers to change will include the effect that any changes would make on his self image as a young 'street-wise' mule, together with his belief about what constitutes acceptable behaviour. Has the service provider any chance of persuading such a person to change his lifestyle?

    c) The risks for Amina are different, in that they are beyond her immediate control: it is her husband who has engaged in risky sex, not her. We know no more about his risks in detail than does Amina.

    Her borriers to change? Clearly, she is financially dependent on her husband. In addition, before deciding on long-term behaviour, she must overcome two major barriers: her shock at discovery of his like behaviour and how this is going to affect her marriage.

d) Tony has not yet been practising risky behaviour, but he has attend the health centre because he is afraid of doing so. Clearly, a cultural or religious practice is the unfortunate cause of his dilemma: the barrier is that he does not wont to offend against this practice.

5. In fact, condoms can provide a number of possible advantages:
   - they prevent transmission of STD, including HIV;
   - they help women to avoid pregnancy;
   - the patient does not need to wait for the STD sores to heal before having sex;
   - women feel dryer inside;
   - the patient will feel safer, with fewer worries;
   - if the patient has to pay for drug treatment, he/she will save money;
   - many men can prolong intercourse if they wear a condom;
   - sheets need washing less often.
6. Many young men might respond as this one does - and some may indeed know how to use condoms correctly. For this reason, it is important to remain tactful; you might respond by accepting his statement and asking him to demonstrate their use to you: 'Fine, why don't you show me (on this model) how you would use one?' This gives you the opportunity to check whether he can use a condom properly and to remind him of the many advantages of doing so. (If, as may be the case, he is too embarrassed to show you, then you could offer to demonstrate it, asking if this is indeed what he would do.)
7. Did you spot the true and false statements? Check your responses against ours below.

   a) Condoms can get *lost inside the woman.*
   False! There is always the slight possibility that, if the man does not use the condom properly, it could slip off before withdrawal, but it could not get lost inside.

   b) *Condoms don 't* protect *against STD including HIV*
   False! Properly-used condoms prevent the transmission of STD including HIV.

   c) *Condoms can be kept in a pocket or wallet indefinitely.*
   Again, false! A wallet or pocket is too warm to store a condom for a long period. Advise patients never to use condoms which are dry, dirty, brittle, yellowed, sticky, melted or damaged.

   d) *It is OK to* use *glycerin or water-based lubricants with condoms.* This one is true! However, remember to advise the patient that it is risky to use grease, oils, lotions or petroleum jelly to make condoms slippery- the oils cause the condoms to break.

e) *Pull the condom tight over the head of the penis to ensure a snug fit. False!* If someone *does* this, the condom *may* burst. *Always leave* space for semen at the tip of the condom.

f) Squeeze *the air out of the tip of the condom as you put it on.* True! This will leave space for the semen to collect.

g) *Condoms should be stored in a cool, dark, dry place. True!* Condoms don't like sunlight, moisture or heat, which is why they don't like living in pockets or wallets too long.

GLOSSARY

Glycerin	Colourless lubricant which is safe to use with condoms
K-YJelly	A jelly-like lubricant which is safe to use with condoms
Oil-based lubricants	Lubricants which are not recommended for use with condoms
Perinatal	Of, or relating to, the time before, during or immediately after childbirth
Petroleum jelly	*Jelly-like* lubricant which is not recommended for use with condoms
Spermicidal foam	Foam which kills sperm, often used as extra protection with condoms
Ulcerative STD	Any STD producing ulcers
Water-based lubricants	lubricants which are also safe to use with condoms
Works	A along term for the equipment that people abusing drugs use to inject themselves

7

PARTNER MANAGEMENT

A. INTRODUCTION

If you have studied Module 5, you will know that partner management is the sixth and final step in educating and supporting patients with STD. Indeed, as we shall show, it is one of the essential components of effective STD case management: one that should be available at any health facility offering STD diagnosis and treatment.

This workbook will help you to offer effective partner management for all your STD patients.

Your learning objectives

This workbook will enable you to:

- explain why partner management is so important;
- anticipate its possible impact on the individuals concerned;
- explore two possible approaches to contacting partners;
- define the issues to discuss with the original patient;
* review the educational and motivational skills you will need when educating STD patients on the need to treat partners;
- treat your patient's partners.

IMPORTANT POINTS

We have already covered basic interpersonal skills in previous workbooks. If you have not already done so, please study these sections first:

- *Sections B and C of Workbook 3, on verbal communication skills;*
- *Section C of Workbook S, on education and motivational skills.*

If you studied Workbooks 3 and 5 some time ago, you might also benefit from a quick review of those sections.

B. PRINCIPLES AND PROBLEMS

This section will enable you to:

- explain why 'partner management' is such an important part of STD case management;
- anticipate its possible impact on the patient and his or her partners;
- apply two key principles to every aspect of partner management;
- compare the costs and benefits of two approaches to contacting partners.

In previous workbooks, we concentrated on the earlier stages of the interview. These included taking the patient's history and examining him or her, making a syndromic diagnosis, and educating the patient on a number of important issues, from complying with treatment to changing their sexual behaviour.

In this module, we cover the final issue to explore with the patient: the need to treat their sexual partners. We will also consider which partners to treat and how to treat them.

QUESTION

1. Why do you think partner management is so important in STD case management? Make a quick note below.:

So partner management helps to break the cycle of STD transmission. Its main features include:

a) treatment of all a patient's sexual partners,
b) for the same STD as the patient, and
c) even if the partners have no sign of STD.

Some clinical research departments study the transmission of STD in order to identify the source of infection. Should we do this? Is it important to do so? Let's consider the issue a moment, with some examples.

A patient we diagnose as having an STD has been infected during unprotected sexual intercourse with one or more infected partners:

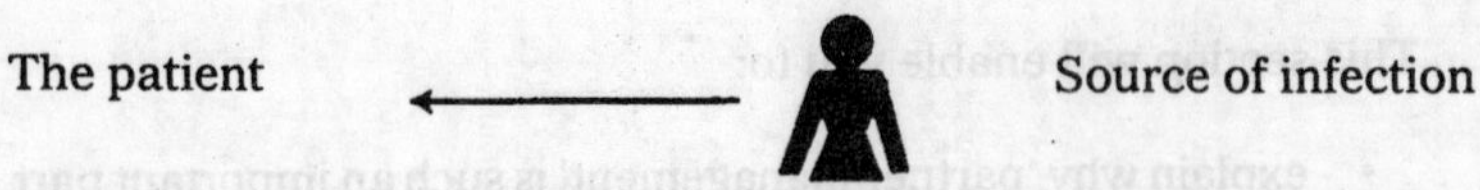

But if the patient has more than one sexual partner, any of these partners could be the source of the infection:

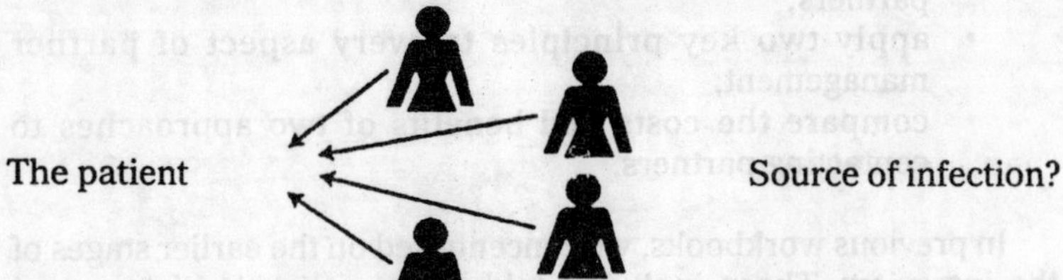

Equally, from the time that the patient was infected with an STD, they have also been infectious: able to transmit the STD infection to other sexual partners. It is often difficult to identify when the patient was infected; for practical purposes, we can assume the period of infectiousness to be two months.

So we must also assume that for two months before the patient come for treatment, all of their sexual partners during that period could have been infected:

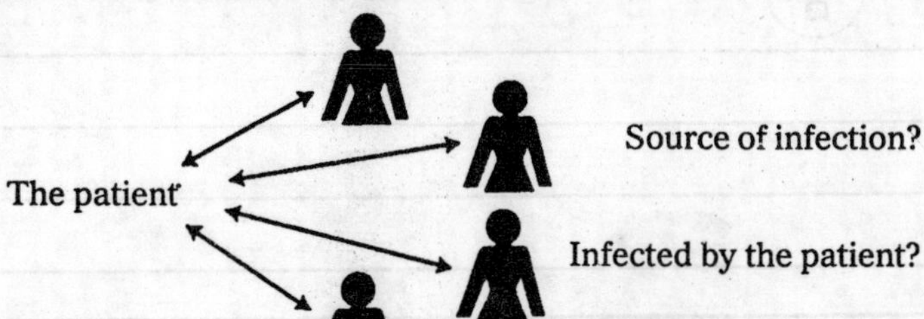

QUESTION

2. *There are only two occasions when it is easy to identify the source of a patient's infection. Can you work out what they are?*

If identifying the source of infection is often difficult or impossible, is it of any value in managing STD cases? No. Identifying the source has no value because our aim is to treat all partners - or all those partners we can reach.

So far, we have identified the three main features of partner management, and we have also stressed the importance of trying to treat and educate all the sexual partners with whom the patient has had unprotected sexual intercourse. Before considering how to manage the treatment of partners, we would like you to consider the possible impact on the individuals concerned.

The impact on individuals

When taking patients' history and educating them, you know the importance of showing respect, responding to emotions and helping patients to overcome barriers and change behaviour. Awareness of having STD can affect a patient's relationships, lifestyle - even their income, as we have discussed in earlier workbooks.

In this final stage of the interview, we must explain to the patient that his or her partners also need to be treated. For many patients this is uncomfortable news. Indeed, it might cause far-reaching damage to the individuals concerned. Why? Please consider the question on the next page.

QUESTION

3. *When might news of STD have a serious affect on the relationship between patient and partner?*

So it is clear that any approach to partner management must take account of the possible impact on the lives of each individual.

QUESTION

4. *What two principles should guide service providers in order ; to protect their STD patients?*

Summary

To be successful in limiting the transmission of STD, any approach to partner management must have these three features:

a) treatment of all a patient's sexual partners,
b) for the same STD as the patient, and
c) even if the partners have no sign of STD.

Partner management must also comply with the principles of confidentiality and non-compulsion: Patients should never be forced to divulge information about partners, and their identity must not be disclosed to anyone outside the health team?

Finally in this section, we will introduce two approaches to partner management and explore how well each approach meets these criteria.

Two approaches to partner management

If the purpose of partner management is to treat as many of the patient's sexual partners as possible, there are two approaches to contacting sexual partners:

- by the patient: this is known as patient referral;
- by a service provider: this is known as provider referral.

Patient referral

In this option it is the patient who takes responsibility for contacting partners and asking them to come for treatment. For reasons we have explained already, many patients might feel unwilling or unable to discuss the STD with partners, so the service provider's aim is to help the patient decide what to do. In fact, a patient might approach partners in several ways:

- by directly explaining about the STD infection and the need for treatment;
- by accompanying a partner to the health centre or asking the partner to attend without specifying why;
- by giving each partner a card asking him or her to attend the centre.

We will explore the practical issues arising from these approaches in Section-C.

Provider referral

This is where the partners of a patient with STD are contacted by a member of the health team - perhaps you or the provider who treated the initial patient, or someone with a particular role connected with searching for and treating partners. The provider asks the partner to attend the clinic for treatment.

Which is the better approach?

On the surface, both approaches to partner management suggest advantages. You might like to spend a few minutes working out what they are, so please try the question here below.

5. *Bearing in mind the two principles of non-compulsion and confidentiality, note down in the box below any possible advantages or disadvantages of each approach that occur to you.*

	Patient referral	*Provider referral*
Advantages		
Disadvantages		

Because of the expense of provider referral and the perceived threat to patient confidentiality, the more practical and workable option is patient referral. This is also the approach recommended by the World Health Organization.

Summary

This first section has set the context and defined two essential principles for partner management. You now know:

- the three main features of partner management;

- why it is such an important part of STD case management;
- its two principles of confidentiality and non-compulsion;
- the two approaches to partner management: provider referral and patient referral, the better of these being patient referral.

In the next section we will develop your understanding of patient referral, exploring the issues to discuss with patients and how to apply your interpersonal skills.

C. PATIENT REFERRAL

The success of patient referral depends on your skills as a service provider: what you say to the patient, how you say it and, equally important, how you listen to the patient and respond to what he or she says. This section will enable you to apply the skills you learned in earlier workbooks to this last and essential objective of treating the patient's partners.

Your learning objectives

This section will enable you to:

- define several issues to explore with the patient;
- review the communication and education skills you need to motivate and support the patient;
- explore the value of referral cards at your health centre.

Educating the patient: the issues

You may remember from Workbook 5 that partner management is the sixth issue on which we need to educate the patient. The service provider needs to:

- explain why it is important for all the patient's partners to be treated;
- remind the patient how to avoid re-infection;
- help the patient decide how to communicate with partners;
- if possible, obtain the names of the patient's partner(s).

To clarify these points, please answer the questions on the next page.

QUESTION

6. *A patient says he'd prefer not to talk to anyone else about his STD infection. He asks "Why do you need to treat my wife and girlfriends?". What would you say to him?*

---

7. *Quick revision for you: what must a patient do in order to avoid being re-infected with the same STD?*

---

8. *We have already said that patients should not be forced to divulge the identity of their partners. When might it be useful to obtain details about their partners?*

Educating the patient: your skills

The skills you need to educate and support the patient about provider referral are exactly the same as for history-taking and for educating the patient on the earlier issues.

Remember that, for the patient, anticipating a talk to partners about STD may provoke feelings as uncomfortable as those the patient first felt when told that he or she had a disease that was sexually transmitted.

Explore how the interview might conclude with them. Read through the first interview and our comments on it, and then try the exercise that follows.

Provider	*John, I said earlier that we'd need to treat your ,girlfriends as well How do you el about talking to them about treatment?*	The service provider starts with an open question in order to find out how John feels and to Identify any
John	*Talk to them about it*	objections to patient referral.
Provider	*You would find it difficult to talk to them?*	Here the service provider is using empathy to encourage John to express his feelings.
John	*Well ...yes...it's one thing to discuss being safe, but it's*	

	something else to ... well to admit to this discharge.	
Provider	*What makes that difficult?*	Open question to probe John's objections further.
John	*They'd say I've been with someone dirty.*	
Provider	*I can understand that that would be difficult for you. But you understood so well how you really got the discharge ... I'm sure you could explain that to your girlfriends.*	The provider is reassuring the patient and reinforcing strengths to help John reel more positive about what he has to do.
John	*What? Explain that anyone can get a sex disease if they sleep with someone without a condom: That it's not about being dirty or anything?*	
Provider	*You're right, it's not. It's just about having unprotected sex with more than one person.*	The provider affirms John's words and offers further explanation to clarify what he has said.
John	*But they haven't got a discharge or anything.*	
Provider	*Women often don't have any symptoms John! but STD can be much more serious for women than for men. I need your help to make sure they do have treatment.*	Explanation is followed by modelling the behaviour that the service provider wants John to adopt.
John	*Yes. So I have to say that...*	

The extract of the interview with John does not illustrate all the skills that the service provider can draw on to use with patients. Try identifying the provider's skills in this extract from the interview with Amina.

QUESTION

9. *Underline anything the provider says that you think illustrates an interpersonal skill, and note what skill you think it is.*

Amina was so shocked by the news of her husband's possible infidelity that she needed time to think about it. Several days later, she has returned; she tells the service provider that she has not had sex and that she is taking the course of tablets correctly but has not yet said anything to her husband. In answer to a question from Amina, her sister-in-law reported hearing that her husband was seen once or twice leaving the bar with a commercial sex worker.

Amina	*I can't say anything to him. He'll blame me I know he will ... I have to think about my family ... he'll blame me even if this disease isn't my fault ...*
Provider	*You're very scared about telling him what you think he's done.*
Amina	*Well . . . yes I am.*
Provider	*I can see you're still very upset about all this, and I sympathies with your position. You've been very wise to come back again to see me and you really want to resolve this and have your husband treated.*
Amina	*But I can't say that to him .*
Provider	*Well, there are two things you could do. You could simply ask him to come to the clinic because he might have your infection, or you could ask someone else to talk to him for you. Which would you prefer?*
Amina	*I could just say that he should come here for a check?*
Provider	*Yes, that's all. I would do the rest. If I gave you this card, could you ask him to bring it with him?*
Amina	*And you would treat him and tell him why he needs it?*
Provider	*I would indeed. What are you going to say to him?*
Amina	*Um. That he might have the same sickness as me, and if he takes that card to the clinic ...*

Notice that the solutions to these two case studies were quite different. In the firsts John was encouraged to speak to his partners himself: something he was willing to do once the provider had helped him resolve the obstacle of embarrassment Many patients will be willing to do the same thing if you educate and support them properly, so patient referral will often be effective.

However, some patients will, like Amina, feel unable to discuss the STD or safe sex with their partners. In this situation, the alternatives of leaving education to the service provider, or of asking a mutual friend or family member to talk to partner, might be equally successful.

We hope that, so for in this section, we have been able to show you how the skills you have already learned for history-taking and education are the same ones you need to discuss patient referral of partners.

In the second case study, the provider offered Amina a card to give to her husband: we will explore the value of such cards next.

Patient referral cards

A young man tells you that a girlfriend asked him to come to the clinic for treatment for an STD. He does not know the name of the syndrome and has no symptoms or signs of any infection. The name he gives for his friend is not in your centre's records, so you have no way to identify what syndrome to treat him for.

Given the high proportion of partners who have no STD symptoms, the above scenario is an example of failed partner management. Without symptoms or stgns of an STD, and with no knowledge of the original patient's syndrome, we cannot treat the patient's partner.

Patient referral cards cn help to resolve this problem and many health centres use them for this purpose. Two examples are illustrated on the next page.

Before turning the page, make a quick note of the information you think a referral card should contain.

Example A

Card No. ________	Card No. ________ Date of Issue: ________
Date of Issue: ________	Issuing Clinic: *Townville, New Town*
Diagnostic Code: ________	Name: ________
Partner's name and details: ________	**Please come to Townville Clinic, bringing this card with you.**
Clinic: *Townville, New Town*	Diagnostic code: ________

The card above has two parts. After writing the necessary details, it is cut along the vertical line and the right side given to the patient to hand to a named partner. The left side is retained for centre records. Cards like this can be linked with the record systems of several different health centres. More importantly, they allow the centre to record the numbers of partners who attend for treatment- as well as the numbers who fail to attend. This would be useful if the centre could contact such partners by provider referral.

Example B

TOWNVILLE CLINIC, TOWNVILLE
Tel- 4S6 834

Opening hours

Monday	9.00 am -	3.00 pm
Tuesday	9.00 am -	3.00 pm
Wednesday	9.00 am -	3.00 pm
Friday	9.00 am -	1.30 pm

9/3/99 *Referral ABC*

This second card is much more simple, yet it contains the information needed to treat a partner. The service provider has merely written the date and a code for the patient's STD syndrome: 'ABC' could be any of the seven STD syndromes. Such a card has the advantage that the patients know it is in general use at the centre, hence no stigma is connected with carrying it. It has no personal details of either the patient or the partner. Disadvantages? None, unless such cards need to be part of an administrative records system, perhaps to monitor the success of patient referral.

To summaries then, a referral card could be extremely useful to help you identify the necessary treatment for anyone who is sent by a patient with STD. The card can contain any extra information that is required, but should never threaten anyone's confidentiality or risk them being stigmotised.

ACTIVITY

With colleagues or your trainer, please discuss any benefits or disadvantages of using referral cards.
Ask if your health centre uses referral cards or plans to do so at some point in the future. If so, how should you use them? What information do they require from the patient? Also make sure that you are familiar with any codes used for the seven STD syndromes.

If referral cards are not used, is there suitable existing literature that could be used instead? What else could you do to increase the frequency of patient referral?

If patient referral fails ...

Provider referral needs special outreach staff who have been specially trained in contacting partners. It is not a viable option for most health centres.

However it might be possible to offer provider referral as a follow-up to patient referral in these two circumstances:

a) when a patient refuses, for whatever reason, to refer partners;
b) when a patient has agreed to refer partners, but they have not since come for treatment.

If the patient refuses to refer partners

If, despite your best endeavors, a patient refuses to refer a partner for treatment provider referral may be the centre's only option.

But perhaps there are still other options open to the service provider? Consider the example below.

One option might be to offer the patient a duplicate course of treatment for a partner. Many service providers would consider this highly inadvisable, arguing that these extra drugs would be sold on the illegal market or otherwise abused, or that more and more patients would demand treatment without prior diagnosis.

On the other hand, some professionals argue that, given the urgency of treating partners, this option can be an effective 'last resort' if practised with caution. They argue that offering a duplicate course of treatment should only be considered when the patient has severe barriers to referring a partner, and when the service provider knows and trusts the patient.

You might like to discuss this idea in more detail with colleagues. Do you consider it viable and, if so, under what conditions?

If a partner fails to come for treatment

In order for your centre to follow up partners who do not come for treatment, the centre would need to have an efficient recording system. After a specific time period - for example, two weeks after the patient was treated - it should be possible to identify those partners who have not been treated so that appropriate arrangements can be made to contact them.

Data may also need to be shared between different clinics. For example, if a female patient's STD is diagnosed during a visit to an antenatal clinic, her partner would probably attend a different clinic for treatment. It would, therefore, be important for outreach service providers to liaisa with all nearby centres offering syndromic diagnosis of STD.

Clearly, there are also implications for the initial interview with the patient. For example, it becomes much more important to obtain the names and details of each partner: where they live or work, and so on. The patient would need reassurance that his or her STD would remain confidential.

Find out whether your health centre has access to any trained outreach staff who could offer provider referral. If necessary, familiarise yourself with the details and procedures to set provider referral in motion.

Summary

This section has explored patient referral in some detail. By now, you should be able to:

- list three issues on which you need to educate the patient;
- identify when it is useful to obtain the names and details about the patient's partners;
- use your education and support skills to communicate effectively;
- if relevant:
  - use referral cards effectively;
  - consider partner referral if necessary.

The action plan at the end of the workbook offers you the opportunity to practise this final part of the patient interview. You might like to practise the skills before moving on to Section-D.

D. TREATING PARTNERS

This short section is about treating the partners of any patient who has been diagnosed as having an STD. How does STD management differ when treating the partner? Is it necessary to examine the partner, and for what STD should we treat him or her? These are the questions you will be able to answer by the end of the section.

QUESTION

10. A young woman tells you that her boyfriend suggested she get a check-up at the health centre. She hands you a card on which you notice that the code for genital ulcer has been written.

a) For what should you treat the young woman?

b) Should you also examine her? Why or why not?

From our answer to question 10, you now know that the aim of partner management is to treat any partner for the same STD as the original patient. To repeat the second answer, examining the patient is not essential, though either you or the patient might prefer to check for other signs.

Otherwise, we deal with the partners of patients in exactly the same way as you have learned to do with the original or 'index' patient, taking their history, treating and educating them and managing their partners.

On the next page is a chart confirming that the partner is treated for the same STD as the patient.

Syndrome of Index patient	Treatment of partner
Urethral discharge	Treat partner for gonorrhoea and chlamydia
Genital ulcer	Treat partner for syphilis and chancroid
Vaginal discharge: Patient treated fcr vaginitis and cervicitis	Treat partner for gonorrhoea and chlamydia
Patient treated for vaginitis only	Not necessary for the partner to be treated unless the discharge is recurrent
Pelvic inflammatory disease	Treat partner for gonorrhoea and chlamydia
Scrotal swelling	Treat partner for gonorrhoea and chlamydia
Inguinal bubo	Treat partner for lymphogranuloma venereum
Neonstal can junctivitis	Treat both parents for gonorrhoea and chlamydia

IMPORTANT POINTS

Notice that, if a female patient with vaginal discharge is diagnosed syndromically as having vaginitis only, her partner does not need to be treated unless the vaginitis is recurrent.

Summary

In this section, you have learned that:

- the partner should be treated for exactly the some STD as the patient, with the proviso linked to vaginal discharge;

- it is not essential to examine the partner;
- history-taking education and partner management are otherwise the same; whether treating original patient or partner.

Do remember to maintain the patient's confidentiality when talking to his or her partner.

E. REVIEW

Now that you have completed Workbook 6, you should be able to:

- explain why partner management is so important;
- anticipate its possible impact on the individuals concerned;
- compare the relative benefits of patient referral and provider referral;
- define four issues to discuss with the original (or index) patient;
- review the educational and motivational skills you will need when educating STD patients on the need to treat partners;
- treat your patient's partners, maintaining each person's confidentiality.

All that remains is the essential task of practising what you have learned. Please turn to the Action Plan next, if you have not already done so.

F. ACTION PLAN

In Workbook 5 you practised how to educate and support your STD patients. This action plan will enable you to refine your skills in the final part of the interview: arranging partner management.

If you are working with a group of people as part of a course, your trainer will guide the role play and explain what you have to do.

If you are studying on your own, you can either:

a) work on this role ploy with the same people as before, completing the roleplay interviews you began with Workbook 5. Each of you should play the some 'patient' as before, and begin the interview where you left off (this should be after demonstrating the use of condoms and gaining the patient's commitment to safe sexual behaviour);

b) work on the role play with different colleagues from before. In this instance, you might prefer to work on a more complete interview, starting either taking the patient's history or simply on the complete education and support of the patient after diagnosis.

On the next few pages are two sets of case studies: the ones used in the action plans in Workbook and a fresh set of four cases.

The patient's role

Please refresh your memory of what happened last time in your interview or select a fresh ones. As before, your aim is to respond as realistically and honestly as you can to whatever the service provider says and does. Don't try and make it either easy or difficult for him or her.

After the role play, you should be the first to give feedback to the service provider. Start by telling him or her how you feel now, at the end of the interview, and review key points during the exercise when the service provider's comments either helped or hindered you in any way.

As the service provider and observer review the exercise, feel free to add any useful insights you have into the service provider's behaviour. At this point, make sure that your suggestions are positive ones that will help the service provider to usefully develop their skills.

The case studies from Workbook 5

Case study 1: Nina

is a 1 9-year-old commercial sex worker who lives in a slum area of town. She has one small child who is often sick. Nina has no partner. She is also using her earnings to help support her family who live in a remote village. Her family disapprove of her job but eagerly accept the money that she sends home. She is afraid of AIDS but finds that many of her clients refuse to use condoms; she also has a limited knowledge about STD. The service provider has diagnosed a genital ulcer; Nina is afraid it might be an STD

Case study 2: John

John is a 24-year-old single man with a good job and his own home. He doesn't want to settle down for a long time, describing himself as 'a good time guy'. He has three sexual partners and sometimes has casual sex too. However, he says he chooses women who are 'clean' or 'married', so he can't understand why he now has a urethral discharge. During the interview he admits that he often gets drunk or injects drugs with one of his partners before sex. The service provider has confirmed the urethral discharge.

Case study 3: Amina

Amina is 35, married with three teenage children. She relies on her husband's income from factory work to support the family. During the interview, she said that she has sex only with her husband. She has already explained that her husband often works late at the factory, and that he go s for a drink with friends occasionally: she can sometimes smell the alcohol on his breath. However she feels quite secure in his faithfulness to her. She came to the centre with no idea of the cause of her abdominal pain - the service provider has diagnosed pelvic inflammatory disease.

Case study 4: Ahmed

Ahmed is 35, married with four children and living in a rural area. He attended an urban clinic with a swelling in his groin which the service provider diagnosed as an inguinal bubo. In answering the service provider's questions, he admitted reluctantly that he has sex with a number of other partners, many of them casual, in the course of his search for work . He regularly travels to the city, working away from home for three months at a time. He says that his wife is currently six months pregnant: he has no been home for two months though he regularly sends home money. He is currently living with a casual partner in the city.

Fresh case studies

Case study 5: Njuguna

Njugana is a 22-year-old single male who lives in the poor area of a large city. He finished secondary school but has been unable to find a steady job in the past three years. He works at whatever causal jobs he can find, trying to save money to start a small business. Most of his friends are in the same situation. They spend their evenings together at one of the local bars. He usually has a few beers and sometimes goes home with one of the young women at the bar. He has had several STD but because they were readily treated at the health clinic, he isn't worried about this urethral discharge.

Case study 6: Pamela

Pamela is a 38-year-oid married woman with four children. She and her family live in a middle class area of the city. Both she and her husband work to put their children through school. Two months ago, Pamela started a sexual relationship with a young male colleague at work. When she noticed her genital ulcer, she felt sure it was punishment for her infidelity and stopped the relationship. She has come to the health centre feeling very guilty and anxious.

Case study 7: Wangui

Wangui is a 1 5-year-old girl, working for her uncle as a housekeeper. Soon after she moved into his house, Wangui was raped by her uncle and since then he has been demanding sex on a regular basis. She tried to run away bock to her family but he caught her and beat her. Her uncle brought her in because she was complaining of lower abdominal pain.

Case study 8: Stephen

At the age of 26, Stephen has finally decided to settle down. He is engaged to a 24-year old teacher, and very much in love. She has asked him to visit the clinic because she thinks he might have an infection. He has handed in a referral card; the code on it indicates that his fiancee has a vaginal discharge, caused by both vaginitis and cervicitis.

The service provider's role

As with Workbook 5, your aim is to obtain feedback on your present skills and areas that you might usefully rehearse or refine.

During the role play, use the same skills as before to persuade and support the patient to refer his or her partners for treatment.

You might like to read the next page, so that you can be sure what the observer is looking for.

After the role play, allow the patient to give you feedback on how he/she felt during the interview. Next, give your own views and feelings about how the education process went. Finally, the observer will provide feedback based on the checklists he or she is using. Feel free to ask either the patient or observer to clarify what they have said: you want to finish the role play with helpful objectives and, hopefully, confirmation of your perceived strengths.

The observer's role

Your aim is to observe this final part of the interview very carefully so that you can provide the 'service provider' with clear, objective feedback on what they have achieved.

Read through the checklist on the next page to familiarise yourself with the skills and issues that the service provider should use.

Time the interview, stopping it after four minutes if it is just about partner management, but allowing fifteen minutes for a complete interview.

As you observe, make quick notes on the skills you see the service provider use and how effectively you think he/she uses them.

Ask the patient, and then the service provider to review the interview first. Start your feedback by responding briefly to the service provider's self-criticism, and then give your feedback, skill by skill or however else you think appropriate. Be willing to give negative criticism if necessary, but offer it in a constructive way, as you did before. Always stress the provider's positive achievements and be as practical as you can.

Finally, lead a discussion about what the three of you have learned from the role ploy. There might be a number of valid issues that this workbook has not included .

Observation Checklist

To what extent does the service provider:

---

a) Deal with partner management issues?

1. The need for partners to be treated
2. How the patient will communicate with partner(s)
3. What the patient could tell his/ her partners) about STD
4. Use of referral card if appropriate

b) Use appropriate education and motivation skills?

1. Explanation and instruction
2. Modelling
3. Reinforcing strengths
4. Exploring choices
5. Rehearsing decisions
6. Confirming decisions

c) Apply communication skills?

1. Facilitation
2. Summarising and checking
3. Reassurance
4. Direction
5. Empathy
6. Partnership

G. ANSWERS

1. Partner management is so important because its purpose is to break the cycle of STD transmission, by treating and educating both the patient and his or her sexual partners. Notice that

partners are treated for the same STD as the patient. Also, partners are treated whether or not they have signs of STD - ensuring that even those people who are asymptomatic are treated.

. In fact, only in these two cases is it possible to identify the source of an STD infection:

- when the patient has had unprotected sexual intercourse with only one other person in the last two months - that person is the source of their infection;
- when the patient is a baby with neonatal can junctivitis - the mother being the source of the infection.

3. News of STD can be especially damaging when a patient or partner hears of their partner's infidelity for the first time. Equally, someone with mistaken ideas about the cause of STD may respond in ways that are inappropriate or extreme. Patients are sometimes blamed for being the source of infection when, as we have seen, it is rarely possible to identify the source of infection.
   Such events might lead to marital breakdown, divorce, loss of home or livelihood, or even ostracism from the social group. You might like to discuss this matter in more detail with your colleagues or trainer.
4. The two principles we were thinking of are that partner management must be confidential and voluntary. The privacy of both patients and partner must be maintained and no-one should be forced to say or do anything they are unwilling to do. These two principles are crucial to any approach to partner management.
5. Your answers to this question may be different from ours, especial if your health centre already uses one or both approaches. If so, please use our notes on the next page as a basis for discussion.

	Patient referral	Provider referral
Advantages	The patient has control over decisions - so both confidential and voluntary. No cost to the health centre	If successful, able to contact and treat more partners more efficient.
Disadvantages	Depends on willingness of patient to refer partners may require	Depends on willingness of Patient patient to divulge

support from service provider.	names. Cost, time and practical problems of tracing partners. Need for extra, highly trained outreach staff. May be viewed by patients as a threat to confidentiality.

Perhaps you agree that the most difficult part of this question was to find positive advantages for provider referral. At a price, provider referral can contact and treat more partners - but at the possible expense of confidentiality. Why? Finding partners can be difficult - even when their name is known. Also, providers trying to find someone may quickly become known in any tight-knit community. Then there is the matter of paperwork: great care must be taken to ensure that such paperwork protects the patient's identity. For all these reasons, we hope you agree that patient referral is the better approach for partner management.

6. In fact you might give any of these reasons why partners must be treated:
   - first, anyone with whom the patient has had unprotected sex in the lust two months may have been infected by the same STD;
   - a partner may be infected even though they have no symptoms,
   - until partners are treated, they risk infecting anyone with whom they have unprotected sex. This includes the risk of re-infecting the patient;
   - women also risk very serious complications if an STD is not treated.

7. This should not have been too difficult. To avoid re-infection, a patient should:

   - avoid having sex until they and their sexual partners have completed a course of treatment for the STD;
   - afterwards, use a condom or practise non-penetrative sex or have sex with only one faithful partner.

8. Knowing the identity of a patient's partners:
   a) is essential only if you need to use provider referral because the patient refuses to make contact with them. But remember that, even in this situation, the patient should not be forced to divulge names indeed, the patient may not know the name or whereabouts of a casual partner;

b) may be useful for any internal records you may keep at the centre. For example, if a patient has asked partners to 'drop by' the health centre without specifying why, records might be the only way to identify what syndrome to treat the partner for - especially if the partner is asymptomatic.

9. We hope that you found this revision helpful. Our notes below explain the skills we think that the service provider is using. Please discuss your analysis with colleagues or your trainer if there is anything you are not sure about.

Amina	*I can't say anything to him. He 'll blame me I know he will ...I have to think about my family...he '11 blame me even if this disease isn 't my fault*	
Provider	*You're very scared about telling him what you think he s done.*	Here the provider checks that she understands Amina's feelings.
Amina	*Well . . . yes I am.*	
Provider	*I can see you're still very upset about all this, and I sympathies with your position. You've been very wise to come back again to see me and you really want to resolve this and have your husband treated.*	The provider offers empathy Reinforcing strength: by praising Amina for her wisdom and understanding of STD, the provider helps her to feel more positive about dealing with it.
Amina	*But I can't SAY that to him*	
Provider	*Well, there are two things you could do. You could simply ask him to come to the clinic because he might have your infection, or you could ask someone else to talk to him for you. Which would you prefer?*	Exploring choices to help Amina select the most appropriate solution.
Amina	*I could just say that he should come here for a check?*	
Provider	*Yes, that's all. I would do the rest. If I gave you this card, could you ask him to bring it with him?*	The provider offers partnership in order to resolve the problem.
Amina	*And you would treat him and tell him why he needs it*	
Provider	*I would indeed. What are you going to say to him?*	The service provider helps Amina to
Amina	*Um. That he might have the*	

	same sickness as me, and if he takes that card to the clinic ...	rehearse what she will say. In this way, she anticipates the real moment when she will speak to her partner.

1 Oa. As with any partner, the young woman should be treated for the some STD as her boyfriend, the original patient. In this case, he had a genital ulcer, so she must also be treated for genital ulcer.

1 Ob. Should this young women be examined? In fact, examination not necessary because you intend to treat her 'n any case. However, you might consider it important to check for signs of other STD. Also, the patient may prefer to be examined ...

GLOSSARY

Index patient	A term used to distinguish between the original patient treated and any partners who are treated. Notice that a partner would become the index patient for any of his or her other partners who are treated
Patient referral	The WHO-recommended method of contacting sexual partners which relies on the patient informing them
Patient referral card	A card the patient can give to sexual partners that might also be part of a health centres's administrative records
Period of infectiousness	The period of time since the patient was infected with an STD and before they are treated. For partner management purposes this can be assumed to be two months
Provider referral	Method of contacting sexual partners which relies on specially trained service providers to do so

8

RECORDING

A. INTRODUCTION

This final workbook is in two parts. The first is about 'recording' STD, while the second is a Development Plan to help you apply all the skills and knowledge that you have learned while studying syndromic case management of STD.

By 'recording' we mean keeping a record of the number of patients we treat who have an STD. As we hope to show in this short workbook, effective recording has important benefits, both for your national ministry of health as well as for your health centre and health district or region.

Your health centre may already be using some sort of recording sheet - in many countries, for example, a simple 'tally' sheet is used to record the number of patients treated for specific diseases. This workbook will help you understand how to use tally sheets and, if appropriate, how to adapt them to collect different sorts of data.

Your learning objectives

This workbook will enable you to:

- explore the possible benefits and limitations of recording, both locally and regionally or nationally;
- identify valid objectives for local or regional recording;
- compare different sorts of tally sheet;
- review any recording systems currently in use in your health centre;
- if appropriate, make STD recording a regular routine as part of your work with patients.

B. RECORDING: WHAT, WHY AND HOW?

The aim of this first section is to explore the benefits and limitations of recording data about STD patients. We need to begin by asking what information we can collect easily, without compromising patients' privacy. After that we will help you to consider how to interpret such data and identify the benefits of doing so.

Clearly, to be successful, any recording system must be accurate. In turn, this means that it must be something all service providers can easily incorporate into their doily routine.

The section will enable you to:

- identify the range of data that can be collected by simple recording methods;
- review the limitations of any interpretation of such data;
- analyse how findings could benefit health services locally as well as regionally and nationally.

What delta can we collect?

We have already stressed that, to be easy to use, tally sheets must not be complicated, so this is a key limitation on the amount of data that anyone outside a research establishment can record. Tally sheets provide bare figures on the numbers of people treated for specific pathologies. The choices include:

- defining the range of pathologies or syndromes to be recorded. A number of countries record all important pathologies: in these, there may be only one reference to 'STD', so that it is not possible to distinguish between different STD. Others may record specific STD by their etiology or syndrome: we will explore their relative merits in Section C.
- defining the populations to be recorded. For STD, this might be all patients attending for treatment, all STD patients treated or more detailed categories of patient, for example by sex and/or age.

What can we learn from such data?

Workbook 1 asked you to consider the value of STD statistics, both international and local to your region. Here we review the limitations of interpreting recorded data, so that we can go on to define some legitimate uses - and their benefits afterwards. To draw on what you learned with Workbook 1, please answer these three questions.

1. *Data collected over the last two years shows there has been a significant increase in the number of patients treated for genital ulcers. What can we interpret this to mean?*

The answer to this first question is more difficult than it seems at first. *You might like to read our comments on page 16 before trying the next two questions.*

2. *Figures for the number of STD cases treated are much lower in Region A than in all other regions. What might this mean?*

3. *Figures show a national decrease in the total number of STD cases treated over the last two months. What might this mean?*

To summaries the outcomes of this exercise, we cannot use the figures from recording to derive causes, nor can we compare them between different centres or regions with any validity. To do either would require more sophisticated epidemiological research.

So how can we interpret the findings of recording? Well, depending on the nature of the data we record, we can work out the frequency and incidence of STD.

> *Frequency: the number of infections over a given time period.*
> *Incidence: the frequency of new infections, expressed as a proportion of the population at risk.*

In other words, recording enables us to define both the number of patients tresteci for STD and what proportion they are of ail patients treated. We can go one step further and define the proportion of STD patients who had a particular syndrome - if we have recorded the appropriate data.

Can we also define the prevalence of STD? First we need to define this term:

> *Prevalence: the proportion of a defined population with the infection at a given point or period in time.*

No, we can't use recording to deduce the prevalence of STD, for two reasons. First, prevalence is usually used to refer to a proportion of the entire population of a country, whereas incidence can be defined in any size of population from nation down to health centre. Secondly, given that successful syndromic case management of STD will treat each patient with STD at their first visit to a health centre, incidence and prevalence would be much the same at health-centre level.

---

4. *To consider the uses and benefits of recording, please try these two questions:*

a) *If recording could provide regular data on the frequency and incidence of STD syndromes, how could your health centre put that information to good use?*

b) *How could such data benefit the region or country's health service?*

Summary

Recording the number of patients that you treat for STD can help your health centre identify trends in the frequency and incidence of STD. In turn this can help the centre plan human and material resources more effectively.

Remember that recording alone cannot explain the distribution or causes of an infection: beware of explaining the reasons for trends or variation without appropriate epidemiological research.

We hope that, by the end of Section-C, you will agree that recording with tally sheets is simple and easy to incorporate into your own work, and that you will be committed to keeping accurate and complete records!

C. USING TALLY SHEETS

Having considered how recording could help us understand the frequency and incidence of STD, we now turn to the main tool for recording: the tally sheet.

Service providers already have many important demands on their time. They need a recording system that is both quick and easy to use, one that will fit easily into the routine between interviewing patients and will not interfere with other work. It must also maintain the confidentiality so important to STD patients. Tally sheets meet these demands.

This section will enable you to:

- compare the value of different sorts of tally sheet;
- learn how to complete a tally sheet if you have not used one before.

Comparing different tally sheets

Tally sheets can be designed to collect a range of data. On the next two pages are a couple of examples for you to look at. Both have been completed by a service provider: the first by making a short vertical mark for each STD patient treated, and the second by crossing through a circle for each patient.

QUESTION

5. *As you look at the two tally sheets, consider these questions:*

   a) *Which tally sheet would enable users to collect more information about STD patients? Why?*

---

b) *Should the tally sheet list STD by pathology or syndrome? Why?*

Tally sheet-example 1

DISEASE NEW CASES	DAYS OF THE WEEK 1	2	3	4	5	6	7	Totals
Accidents	111		11		11	1	1	
Acute poliomyelitis					1			
Anaemia	1		1		1			
Bilharzia	1		111	11	11	1	1	
Catarac.						1		
Chicken pox								
Diarrhoeal diseases	111	11111	11	111	1111	111		
Gonorrhoea			11			1	1	
Guinea worm	1			1				
Hypertension			1					
Infectious hepatitis								
Intestinal worms	1	1			1	1		
Leprosy								
Malaria			1		1			
Total New Cases								
Re-attendances								
Referrals								

Tally Sheet- example 2

CLINIC: ----------------	NAME OF OFFICER: ------------------
ADDRESS: ----------------	POSITION: ------------------
DATE: ----------------	SIGNATURE: ------------------

SYNDROME	TALLY				TOTAL CASES
	10 – 19	20 – 29	30 – 39	40+	
MALES Urethral discharge	00000 00000	ØØØ00 00000	Ø0000 00000	Ø0000 00000	
Genital ulcers	ØØ000 00000	Ø0000 00000	Ø0000 00000	ØØ00 00000	
Scrotal swelling	ØØ00 00000	00000 00000	00000 00000	00000 00000	
Inguinal bubo	00000 00000	Ø0000 00000	00000 00000	Ø0000 00000	
TOTAL MALES					
FEMALES Vaginal discharge	00000 00000	00000 00000	ØØØØ0 00000	ØØ000 00000	
Genital ulcers	00000 00000	Ø0000 00000	ØØ000 00000	00000 00000	
Lower abdominal pain	Ø0000 00000	ØØØØ0 00000	ØØ000 00000	ØØ000 00000	
Inguinal bubo	00000 00000	00000 00000	Ø0000 00000	00000 00000	
TOTAL FEMALES					
TOTAL BY AGE					
Neonatal conjunctivitis	00000 00000			**GRAND TOTAL**	

In the answer to question 5, we suggest that the tally sheet above enables users to record a useful range of data for each STD syndrome. However, if this means that service providers need to use two tally sheets - one for general pathologies and one for STD syndromes - there is a much greater risk of errors in the data collected. Health centres should balance very carefully the value of specific data and the complexity of recording.

How to complete a tally sheet

The rest of this section will help you to understand how to read and use tally sheets if you have not done so before.

ACTIVITY

6. To help you practise reading tally sheets, answer the questions below by referring to Tally Sheet 2 opposite.

a) How many males were treated for urethral discharge?

---

b) How many females of 30 or over were treated for vaginal discharge?

---

c) How many people were treated for genital ulcers?

---

d) How many males between 20-29 have been treated for any STD?

---

e) How many people of 40 or over have been treated?

Now that you understand how the tally sheet details are recorded, it is time to practise using a tally sheet yourself. This is important if you have never used one before.

QUESTION

7. Try completing the blank tally sheet on the next page by recording all the people below.:

a) During the course of a week, you treat all the STD cases below. Please record them in the appropriate boxes on the tally sheet.
b) Then total each column and row.

Urethral discharge:
4 males aged 18, 22, 24 and 45.
Vaginal discharge:
5 females aged 15, 17, 21, 24 and 32.
Genital ulcers:
3 males aged 19, 21 and 24.

2 females aged 19 and 20.

Lower abdominal pain:

2 females aged 18 and 35

Inguinal bubo:

1 male aged 22.

Tally sheet 3

CLINIC: _______________		NAME OF OFFICER: _______________		
ADDRESS: _______________		POSITION: _______________		
DATE: _______________		SIGNATURE: _______________		

SYNDROME	TALLY				TOTAL CASES
	10 – 19	20 – 29	30 – 39	40+	
MALES Urethral discharge	00000 00000	00000 00000	00000 00000	00000 00000	
Genital ulcers	00000 00000	00000 00000	00000 00000	00000 00000	
Scrotal swelling	00000 00000	00000 00000	00000 00000	00000 00000	
Inguinal bubo	00000 00000	00000 00000	00000 00000	00000 00000	
TOTAL MALES					
FEMALES Vaginal discharge	00000 00000	00000 00000	00000 00000	00000 00000	
Genital ulcers	00000 00000	00000 00000	00000 00000	00000 00000	
Lower abdominal pain	00000 00000	00000 00000	00000 00000	00000 00000	
Inguinal bubo	00000 00000	00000 00000	00000 00000	00000 00000	
TOTAL FEMALES					
TOTAL BY AGE					
Neonatal conjunctivitis	00000 00000			**GRAND TOTAL**	

Finally, in this section, here is an outline of a typical recording procedure within a health centre:

1. At the start of a week or month, each service provider starts a fresh fully sheet, recording each patient treated for STD as the tally sheet requires.

2. At the end of the week or month, a designated provider or clerk collects the tally sheets and collates the data.
3. The data is stored and interpreted, then made available to staff at the centre. It may also be sent to the Ministry of Health's epidemiology unit.
4. At the epidemiology unit, all data received is compiled and distributed in periodic reports.

The assignment will ask you to check what happens to any data collected by your own health centre.

D. REVIEW

We hope you now understand why recording is so important, and how easy it will be to incorporate an STD tally sheet into your working routine.

Without accurate records, your country, region or even your health centre will be unable to monitor trends in the STD epidemic. More importantly, it may not be possible to plan sufficient facilities and drugs for future treatment. Nor will you have enough data to decide whether your treatment, education or partner management techniques are effective.

If your health centre uses any recording system, your role in recording is a vital one. Always use the tally sheets carefully and accurately to help your clinic make its STD care as effective as possible.

To conclude this workbook, please turn to the assignment on the next page. It will help you to:

- review any recording systems currently in use in your health centre;
- if appropriate, make STD recording a regular part of your routine at work.

E. ASSIGNMENT

Please work through this assignment with the help of your trainer or supervisor.

Does your health centre use tally sheets or any other recording methods? If so, please work through the questions and ideas below. If not, please consider the questions on the next page.

1. What recording methods does your health centre currently use?
2. a) How effective is each method?
   b) Would it enable you to monitor trends in the frequency of STD syndromes or their incidence in your centre's patient population?
   c) How can the data it provides be used locally?
   d) What other data might you usefully collect?

3. Plan how you will fit using tally sheets or other recording methods into your daily schedule.

These questions might help you plan.

a) Where are the tally sheets stored?
b) Who collects them from you, and when?
c) Where can you keep the tally sheet when you are working? (It must be within easy reach and visible so that you don't forget it!)

4. If necessary, learn how to use the recording method, perhaps by practising with a colleague as we have done with you. For example, you could take turns to call out imaginary patients (for example, 'a 16-year old male with a genital ulcer') and see how accurately you keep record what the other says.

The success of your health centre's recording depends on everyone recording accurately. Make sure recording fits in well with the rest of your STD case management. If you feel comfortable using it, your tally sheets will be accurate.

If your health centre does not currently use any recording methods, perhaps you could help develop a simple tally sheet, for use on a trial basis. If so:

1. Agree the objective of the recording. This might be, for example, to monitor the frequency of patients treated for each STD syndrome per week or month. You might also want to break those figures down by sex and or age: agree objectives suitable for your locality.
2. Design a simple tally sheet that service providers could use easily.
3. Find out who will collect the tally sheets and compile the data from them.
4. Plan how each service provider will be kept up to date on trends from month to month.

F. ANSWERS

1. The aim of these three questions is to explore the limitations of interpreting STD data. We must apologise for question 1 because, in fact, it is misleading - for reasons we will explain in a moment.

At face value, a significant increase in the number of patients treated for STD seems to suggest there has been an equal increase in the general population. But the data cannot be interpreted in such a way because these patients may not be a representative sample of the population. To find out the size of the STD epidemic would require research of a different nature. The only sure interpretation of this data would be that more patients have been treated for genital ulcers. Otherwise, we can only suggest possible interpretations based on informed guesses. To name just two:

- introducing quality care for patients with STD should itself have encouraged a significant increase in the number of people who come for treatment - including for treatment of genital ulcers;
- new or improved recording techniques might have lead to more accurate data collection than in the past.

You might like to discuss other possible causes of such an increase with your colleagues or trainer. (By the way, have you worked out why our question was misleading? We asked 'What can we interpret this to mean?' when our question should have been 'What might this mean?'!)

2. Again, comparison of any variation between regions is difficult because there can be so many possible reasons for the variation. For example, it could be that Region A has fewer health facilities than other regions, or that the region is more rural, so that fewer people have access to a facility. Alternatively, the population of Region A might rely more on traditional healers, so that STD patients do not appear in their statistics. You could probably identify a number of equally plausible explanations. Remember that we cannot automatically assume fewer cases treated in Region A to mean there is less STD in the population of Region A than elsewhere.

3. Once again, we cannot infer an automatic explanation for the decrease in the number of patients treated. Variations over time might be caused by seasons patterns such as heavy rains which make travel difficult, or harvesting, which draws people away from villages. They may be caused by other events, such as a new health facility which has attracted patients with STD. If monthly recording data is available, over several years it would be possible to identify any regular seasonal variations in cases treated for STD.

4 a) We can use data on the frequency and incidence of STD to assess trends in the numbers of STD cases we treat. This could help the centre better to plan its human and material resources, such as drugs and, if applicable, condoms. Knowing trends and anticipating seasonal variations may also enable the health centre to plan more relevant campaigns and research projects, perhaps with other services such as community and education centres.

4b) Regional and national health services could also use the data to help plan resources: financial as well as human and material. Equally, they might be able to plan more effective health education campaigns and liaise with other services that could help in the fight against STD.

Also, although we have stressed that we cannot draw conclusions about why variations occur between or within regions or countries, such variation do suggest possible issues that could be researched in more detail. So recording also helps to identify useful research that would add to the understanding of STD epidemiology.

5a) You probably found this question easy to answer, in that example 2 is definitely the more effective tally sheet for recording STD. It enables users to record all seven of the STD syndromes we have included in this programme . In addition, it allows users to record the number of males and females treated for each syndrome, each further subdivided by age.

The first example is less useful simply because it includes in its listing only one STD: gonorrhoea. It could tell us nothing about the frequency of any other STD syndromes. However, such a tally sheet could be usefully adapted for use in a general clinic or health centre. For example, it would enable us to identify the incidence of STD patients among centre users. If such a tally sheet could not list all main STD, it would be better simply to have 'STD' in the 'Disease' column.

5b) Any health centre using the syndromic approach to STD diagnosis should use tally sheets that record STD by syndrome. Why? Because to make a clinical or etiological diagnosis requires sophisticated tests and methods

6. Please check your answers with these below. If you found the exercise difficult, please consult your trainer - but don't worry, there would always be others willing to do this for you if you find maths difficult.

a) 5 }
b) 6 } Each of these figures is derived by reading the table
c) 9 } horizontally.
d) 5 To reach this figure, you read vertically down the 20-29 group for males.
e) 8 To reach this figure, you read vertically down the 40+ age group for both males and females.

7. Your completed tally sheet should look exactly like the one give here below. If you found this exercise at all difficult, please consult a colleague and ask them to help you (it's really very easy once you get the idea). Using tally sheets for recording is much easier at work than it is in this exercise because you only record one person at a time, as you treat him or her

CLINIC: ------------------	**NAME OF OFFICER:** ------------------
ADDRESS: ------------------	**POSITION:** ------------------
DATE: ------------------	**SIGNATURE:** ------------------

SYNDROME	**TALLY**				**TOTAL CASES**
	10 – 19	**20 – 29**	**30 – 39**	**40+**	
MALES Urethral discharge	Ø0000 00000	ØØ000 00000	00000 00000	Ø0000 00000	4
Genital ulcers	Ø0000 00000	ØØ000 00000	00000 00000	00000 00000	3
Scrotal swelling	00000 00000	00000 00000	00000 00000	00000 00000	0
Inguinal bubo	00000 00000	Ø0000 00000	00000 00000	00000 00000	1
TOTAL MALES	2	5	0	1	8
FEMALES Vaginal discharge	ØØ000 00000	ØØ000 00000	Ø0000 00000	00000 00000	5
Genital ulcers	Ø0000 00000	Ø0000 00000	00000 00000	00000 00000	2
Lower abdominal pain	Ø0000 00000	00000 00000	Ø0000 00000	00000 00000	2
Inguinal bubo	00000 00000	00000 00000	00000 00000	00000 00000	0
TOTAL FEMALES	4	3	2	0	9
TOTAL BY AGE	6	8	2	1	17
Neonatal conjunctivitis	00000 00000			**GRAND TOTAL**	17

F. DEVELOPMENT PLAN

This development plan is for you to work through once you have completed your training in STD case management.

The aim of the plan is to enable you to continue reflecting on, and developing, your skills and the service you offer.

Your trainer may ask you to work through this during a training session. Equally you could discuss it with your trainer or supervisor as suggested below:

The plan is in three parts:

Part 1.	Th s first part asks you to reflect on what you have learned, so that you can identify what you can do well, together with any 'weaknesses' things you still want to improve or learn more about.
Part 2.	Next you will be asked to plan how you can develop all the necessory skills, to make sure you give the best possible service to your patients or clients.
Part 3.	And thirdly, you will be able to review your skills again in a month's time. Any new set of complex skills like the ones you have learned takes time to get right, so it is airways worth reviewing what is happening .

1. Reflect on your learning

Please start by flipping back through each of the workbooks you have studied paying particular attention to the workbook objectives and action plans.

Next, answer these questions.

ACTIVITY

What skills do you feel confident that you have learned well, and can now do effectively? This might be anything that pleases you personally in what you have achieved, or that others have praised you for - including your colleagues and patients!

Are there any skills that you feel you have either not understood or not learned sufficiently? Perhaps you have not had enough time to practise with real patients, or colleagues or patients have criticised your work? If so, please note these below:

If you were to ask three patients or clients what they think of your service, what would you like them to say about you?

What do you think your colleagues or patients would actually say about your service? If this is different, why?

Please discuss what you have noted above with your supervisor or trainer. Record any different or extra points they make about either your strengths or your weaknesses.

2. Plan your skills development

Now the important part. We suggest you set yourself some development objectives. These will include continuing the skills you have achieved satisfactorily, and working on anything you want to improve. You might wish to think of it as a learning 'contract'.

I will continue to work to the same high standard in these things:

I intend to develop my skills and/or confidence in the following things:

What I intend to improve:	How I could develop this skill:	Who can help:	My target date:

3. Review your progress

By the time you conduct this review, you should have been working in STD case management for at least a month, whatever your responsibilities.

Please go back over the notes you made for part 2 in this development plan, and note down how you feel you have progressed in both your strengths and weaknesses.

By now you are in a good position to comment on ways you might improve STD management practices at your facility. Yo may have come across issues or problems that you didn't anticipate during the training. There may be difficulties with resources, administration or team-work, or you may have found working with STD patients more stressful or upsetting than you expected.

Please note down:

- *anything that you can resolve or improve personally,*
  and
- *any issues or problems that require the attention of your supervisor or the team.*

____

____

____

____

It is essential to ensure that the whole service works efficiently, so please raise any problems you have noted with your supervisor or other members of your team.

And that completes this development plan. However, it is unlikely to be the end of your self-development. So urgent is the need to counter the STD epidemic that we will always find new challenges to our skills and understanding. The size of the task might seem overwhelming, but you are part of a strategy that is the best one yet devised, and has the greatest chance of success.

We wish you success in your continued endeovours.

GLOSSARY

Workbook 7: Recording

Accredited facilities	All public and private sector health facilities
Epidemiology	The study of the incidence, distribution and causes of an infection or disease in a population
Frequency	The number of infections over a given time period
Incidence	The frequency of new infections, expressed as a percentage of the population at risk
Prevalence	The proportion of a defined population

	with the infection at a given point or period in time. Usually used to refer to the population of a country
Recording	Keeping a record of the number people treated for STD in order to identify the trends in frequency and incidence of STD syndromes
Tally sheet	A chart on which the numbers of patients can be recorded quickly and accurately. The sheet is then used to summaries and collate the data collected
Unaccredited facilities	Traditional healers and drug vendors
Universal reporting	All clinics report the number of cases treated

•••